Ketogenic Diet and Intermittent Fasting for Beginners

A Complete Guide to the Keto Fasting Lifestyle.
Gain the Weight Loss Clarity You Need

Written by Jimmy Clark

© **Copyright 2018 by Jimmy Clark - All rights reserved.**

The following eBook is reproduced below with the goal of providing information that is as accurate and reliable as possible. Regardless, purchasing this eBook can be seen as consent to the fact that both the publisher and the author of this book are in no way experts on the topics discussed within and that any recommendations or suggestions that are made herein are for entertainment purposes only. Professionals should be consulted as needed prior to undertaking any of the action endorsed herein.

This declaration is deemed fair and valid by both the American Bar Association and the Committee of Publishers Association and is legally binding throughout the United States.

Furthermore, the transmission, duplication or reproduction of any of the following work including specific information will be considered an illegal act irrespective of if it is done electronically or in print. This extends to creating a secondary or tertiary copy of the work or a recorded copy and is only allowed with an expressed written consent from the Publisher. All additional rights reserved.

The information in the following pages is broadly considered to be a truthful and accurate account of facts and as such any inattention, use or misuse of the information in question by the reader will render any resulting actions solely under their purview. There are no scenarios in which the publisher or the original author of this work can be in any fashion deemed liable for any hardship or damages that may befall them after undertaking information described herein.

Additionally, the information in the following pages is intended only for informational purposes and should thus be thought of as universal. As befitting its nature, it is presented without assurance regarding its prolonged validity or interim quality. Trademarks that are mentioned are done without written consent and can in no way be considered an endorsement from the trademark holder.

Table of Contents

Introduction 14

Chapter 1: The History and Science Behind the Ketogenic Diet 16

    This History 16

    The Science 23

Chapter 2: The Health Benefits of Going Keto 38

    Weight Loss 38

    Anti-Aging 40

    Parkinson's Disease 41

    Epilepsy 42

    Alzheimer's Disease 44

    Diabetes 46

    High-Cholesterol 48

    Polycystic Ovary Syndrome (PCOS) 50

    Decreased Inflammation 51

    Non-Alcoholic Fatty Liver Disease 51

- Cancer 52
- Multiple Sclerosis 53
- Mood Stabilization 54
- Appetite Control 55

Chapter 3: The Fundamentals of the Ketogenic Diet 57

- The Standard Ketogenic Diet 57
- The Targeted Ketogenic Diet 59
- The Cyclical Ketogenic Diet 61
- The High-Protein Ketogenic Diet 62
- Reaching Ketosis 63
- Stay Hydrated 64
- Refuel on Electrolytes 65
- Eat as Needed 66
- Light Exercise 67
- Sleep Well 67

Chapter 4: What You Can and Cannot Eat 69

- Avocados 70
- Olives 71

Sardines 71

Coconut Oil 72

Walnuts 73

Almonds 74

Pecans 74

Grass-Fed Butter 75

Broccoli 76

Asparagus 77

Zucchini 77

Mushrooms 78

Green Beans 79

Blackberries 80

Strawberries 80

Raspberries 81

Shrimp 82

Grass-Fed Beef 83

Liver 83

Chapter 5: The History and Science Behind Intermittent Fasting 85

The History 85

The Science 91

Increased Growth Hormone 93

Weight Loss 94

Less Muscle Loss 94

Decreases Insulin Resistance 95

Reduces Inflammation 95

Improved Heart Health 96

Delays Aging 98

Induces Cell Repair 98

May Prevent and Treat Cancer 99

Reduces Oxidative Stress 99

Converts Fats 100

Creates More Brain Cells 100

Increases Energy 101

Controls Seizures 102

Boosts Metabolism 102

Chapter 6: The Fundamentals of Intermittent Fasting 103

The Fed and Fasted State 103

12/12 106

16/8 107

Meal Skipping 108

2 Days Every 5 Days 109

Weekly 24-Hour Fast 110

Alternate Day Fasting 111

Warrior Diet 112

Busting the Myths 114

Chapter 7: Combining Intermittent Fasting and the Ketogenic Diet 131

More Manageable Fasting 132

Enter Ketosis Sooner 133

Lose Weight Faster 134

Create a Self-Healing Environment 136

Boost Your Brain 137

Burn More Fat 138

Spend Less Time Cooking 139

Reduce Inflammation and Oxidative Stress

....140

Energy Boost 141

Detox...142

Chapter 8: Common Mistakes and How to Avoid Them 144

Obsessing over the Scale 144

Not Eating Enough.................................... 146

Getting Dehydrated 147

Not Sleeping Enough.................................148

Not Knowing Your Macros........................ 149

Not Eating Enough Protein 150

Avoiding Vegetables 151

Obsessing over Ketone Levels 151

Too Many Nuts and Too Much Dairy........ 153

Eating Low-Carbohydrate Treats.............. 154

Drinking Alcohol 156

Not Planning.. 156

Cheating... 157

Too Much Snacking................................... 158

Not Exercising 159

Doing Too Much Too Soon 160

Giving Up..161

Chapter 9: Planning for Success 163

Chapter 10: Possible Side Effects 168

Headaches 168

Dehydration... 170

Electrolyte Imbalance 171

Fatigue...171

Malnutrition 172

Brain Fog 173

Hunger... 174

Kidney Stones..175

Insomnia.. 176

Bad Breath 178

Muscle Cramps 179

Digestive Problems...................................180

Hair Loss 183

Elevated Heart Rate 184

Ketoacidosis 185

Reduced Exercise Performance 187

Chapter 11: Frequently Asked Questions 189

Is There a Better Time of Day to Fast? 189

Do I Start Counting My Fast After Completing the Meal or After the First Bite? 190

Will I Lose Muscle Tone If I Practice Intermittent Fasting Long-Term? 190

Does 20 Calories of Cream in My Coffee Hurt? 191

Should I Still Fast If I'm at My Goal Weight? 191

Do I Have to Fast Every Day or Is It Okay to Miss Some Days? 192

Is There Any Way to Not Skip Breakfast If Get My Daily Energy from It? 192

How Long Is It Safe to Fast For? 193

Will I Be Hungry While Fasting? 193

How Long Does It Take to Get into Ketosis? 194

Can I Drink While Fasting? 194

Can I Take My Medicine While Fasting? . 195

Why Do I Get Cold While Fasting? 195

Is Intermittent Fasting Safe for Women? 196

Will I Have Cravings? 197

Is the Ketogenic Diet Safe on the Kidneys? 197

Will I Feel Tired and Weak? 198

Is the Ketogenic Diet a Fad? 198

Is The Ketogenic Diet and Fasting Safe During Pregnancy or Breastfeeding? 199

What Is the Difference Between Low-Carbohydrate and the Ketogenic Diet? 199

How Many Carbohydrates Can You Eat and Still Be in Ketosis? 200

Is the Ketogenic Diet Safe for Everyone? 200

Conclusion 202

Introduction

In a world full of crash and fad diets, it can be difficult to know how to lose weight in a healthy and manageable way that will actually keep the weight off. Many diets that claim success may help you drop the pounds, but only leave you weak, exhausted, hungry, and stressed. What is worse is that these crash diets often leave your metabolism a wreck, causing you to soon gain the weight back. They may help you lose weight in the short-term, but they have long-term negative consequences.

Reaching your goals does not have to be such a difficult and stressful process. In this book, you will learn all about how the ketogenic diet and intermittent fasting can help you not only lose the weight but how to lose it in a healthy way that will also keep the pounds off in the long-run.

While crash diets come and go the ketogenic diet has been around, helping people not only lose weight but gain health, for nearly a century. Likewise, intermittent fasting has been around for weight loss, religion, health, and as a necessity for thousands of years. Not only is there an abundance of anecdotal evidence for the health benefits and weight loss effects of the ketogenic diet and intermittent fasting, but there are numerous studies that prove these beneficial effects as well. And, more studies are continuing to come out every day.

By the time you finish this book, you will know everything you need to successfully lose weight with the ketogenic diet and intermittent fasting, whether you need to lose five pounds or even one-hundred pounds.

Chapter 1: The History and Science Behind the Ketogenic Diet

The world has recently been taken by storm by the ketogenic diet and its claims of health and weight loss. The ketogenic diet, or often simply referred to as 'keto diet', is a low-carbohydrate, moderate-protein, and high-fat diet. It may seem contradictory to well-known health recommendations to cut out grains and increase fat, yet, there are numerous studies showing the health benefits of this plan. The ketogenic diet is not just another crash diet scheme; it is a long-term plan for health, wellness, and yes, weight loss.

This History

While the ketogenic diet would not originate

until the 1920s, the groundwork for it began back in 1911 when the first modern study on fasting for the treatment of epilepsy was conducted in France. In this study twenty different epileptic patients of various ages went on a low-calorie vegetarian diet, paired with periods of fasting. While most of the patients struggled under the strenuous restrictions of this diet, two of them did benefit enormously. These patients experienced a remarkable improvement in their mental capabilities, quite a contrast to their medication which had dulled their minds.

Around the same time, Bernarr Macfadden, an American advocate of physical culture, which is a method of combining diet and strength training, began popularizing fasting for health. Of Macfadden's supporters, a doctor of osteopathic medicine, Hugh Conklin, began to treat his hundreds of epileptic patients with fasting. Conklin would recommend his patients maintain an eighteen to twenty-five-day fast, to rid the body of supposed toxins. While he only had a fifty percent success rate in adults, Conklin was able to successfully treat ninety percent of the children under his care. Overall twenty percent of Conklin's patients were able to become seizure-free, and fifty percent had some improvement. Conklin's treatment was so successful that it soon became a mainstream treatment by neurologists.

Dr. McMurray wrote to the New York Medical Journal in 1916, claiming success in treating epileptic patients beginning in the year of 1912 with a fast followed with a sugar and starch-free diet. Soon thereafter, once seeing Conklin's success first-hand, a prominent endocrinologist, Dr. H. Rawle Geyelin of the New York Presbyterian Hospital decided to try to recreate the outcome in the treatment of his own thirty-six patients. Geyelin reported his success to the American Medical Association. Studies continued into the 1920s. The parents of one of Conklin's successfully treated patients, Charles Howland, gave his brother, John Howland, a professor of pediatrics at Johns Hopkins Hospital, $5,000 in order to continue the research of ketosis and epilepsy. This payment was able to fund research by neurologist Stanley Cobb and his assistant, William G. Lennox.

In the year of 1921 endocrinologist, Dr. Rollin Woodyatt found that water-soluble compounds, acetone, acetoacetate, and β-hydroxybutyrate were produced by the liver, as a result of starvation, fasting, and in a diet both high in fat and low in carbohydrates. These compounds are known as ketones.

During the same year Dr. Russell Wilder, from the Mayo Clinic, gave this diet the name it is now known for. Dr. Wilder proposed that a ketogenic diet could be equally as effective in treating epilepsy, but with the ability to be maintained for much longer periods of time.

Another doctor at the Mayo Clinic, Dr. Peterman, treated his patients following the diet and noted improvements in their behavior and cognitive function. Dr. Peterman believed and stressed the importance of teaching caregivers how to manage the diet, individualizing the plan for each patient, and close continuous follow-ups. Before long the success of the ketogenic diet become well-known, and it was recorded in nearly every comprehensive textbook on childhood epilepsy between the years of 1941 and 1980.

In 1938, Tracy J. Putnam and H. Houston Merritt made a historic discovery of an anticonvulsant drug, Dilantin, which became a pioneer in epileptic drug research and therapy. However, this new era in drug treatment led to a decline in the use and knowledge of the ketogenic diet.

Due to the decline of the use of the ketogenic

diet in 1971 Dr. Peter Huttenlocher, from the University of Chicago, introduced medium-chain triglycerides, otherwise known as MCTs, into the ketogenic diet. It had been found that MCTs produce more ketones per unit of energy than other sources of fat, meaning that patients on the diet were able to increase their protein and carbohydrate levels compared to the original version of the diet. This enabled epileptic children to enjoy a wider range of more palatable foods while on the diet, which made it easier to maintain.

Despite Dr. Huttenlocher's efforts, the ketogenic diet continued to decline as a wider variety of anticonvulsants became available. Many doctors believed that anticonvulsants were the wave of the future and that the ketogenic diet would no longer be necessary or justified. This led to fewer epileptics being placed on the diet and a decrease in dietitian awareness. As there were fewer dietitians fully aware of the ketogenic diet it would often be implemented incorrectly with miscalculations, leading people to believe that the diet was unhealthy and ineffective.

It took over two decades but the ketogenic diet began to make a comeback when it was discovered that it could be used to treat epilepsy that is resistant to drug therapy. The beneficial effects of the ketogenic diet made national attention when NBC's series Dateline aired a program in October of 1994 reporting on the case of Charlie Abrahams, the son of Hollywood producer Jim Abrahams. Charlie, a two-year-old, lived with epilepsy that was uncontrolled by either mainstream or alternative treatments until his parents learned of the ketogenic diet and brought Charlie to John Freeman at John's Hopkins Hospital, which was one of the few hospitals to continue in the treatment of epilepsy with the ketogenic diet.

Once on the ketogenic diet, Charlie made a

rapid recovery and resumed to make developmental progress, which inspired his parents to create the Charlie Foundation in order to fund further research and promote the diet. Abrahams even produced a movie which aired on TV in 1997 starring Meryl Streep, *First Do No Harm*.

A multicenter prospective study on the ketogenic diet began in 1994, and the results were shared with the American Epilepsy Society two years later and in 1998, the results were officially published. This lead to an explosion of scientific interest in the ketogenic diet and studies continued to follow.

The Science

The human body is capable of transmuting any type of ingested nutrient into a usable energy source. Fats, proteins, and carbohydrates can all be converted into fuel through various metabolic processes. This means that the process of ketosis is natural and something the body can go through on a daily basis without a person even realizing it. Whenever you do not have glucose readily available to use as fuel because you skipped a meal, exercised for over an hour, or ate a low number of carbohydrates that day, you can unknowingly slip into a light ketosis.

But first, to understand how ketones are made you need to know how the body processes carbohydrates. After eating a high-carbohydrate meal or excessive amounts of proteins, the metabolic process will break it down into a simple sugar, known as glucose, as this will provide cells with the quickest source of adenosine triphosphate, or rather ATP energy. ATP is a complex organic chemical that is the primary molecule used to provide energy to nearly every cell and system in the body.

Every type of fuel, whether fat, carbohydrate,

or protein can increase your body's ATP levels to some extent. The body uses much of this energy solely to maintain itself every day, yet, in today's age, many people consume highly processed and high caloric foods without expending the energy needed to burn off all of those extra calories. Rather than excreting the excess calories the body will store it in case of emergency, and it does this in two ways:

1. **Glycogenesis:** During the process of glycogenesis any excess glucose is converted to glycogen, which is the stored version of sugar that is kept in the liver and muscles. The body can store approximately two-thousand calories of glycogen between both the muscles and liver. Depending on the person and their energy output this glycogen can be depleted within six to twenty-four hours when no other calories are consumed during that time.

There is another source of energy storage that will help sustain us when we run out of glycogen, which is the process of lipogenesis.

2. **Lipogenesis:** Once there is no more space for glycogen stores in your muscles and liver, any extra glucose will be converted through a process known as lipogenesis. This process converts glucose into fat and stores it as adipose, also known as body fat. This type of storage, unlike glycogenesis, is unlimited and has the ability to sustain us for months with a limited food supply.

Whether nutrients are from carbohydrates, fats, or proteins, the human body can use it as fuel. A large majority of the body's cells, those with mitochondria, are able to utilize fat as an energy source, which has quite a few benefits. Yet, there are some cells in the body that are not able to burn fat, these cells being red blood cells, brain cells, testicle cells, and kidney medulla. Thankfully, these cells are not deprived of their important fuel on the ketogenic diet, as once your body burns through any glycogen you have stored a process called gluconeogenesis begins. Due to the gluconeogenesis process, our bodies will turn lactate, glycerol, and amino acids into glucose to fuel the cells that require it to function.

While gluconeogenesis is a powerful ability, it would also be a double-edged sword if it were not paired with the liver's ability to produce ketones as an energy source. This is because the amino acids that the gluconeogenesis turns into glucose are protein, and if you are not eating enough it will take the amino acids from your muscle mass, causing you to lose strength and energy. If not for the liver producing ketones as fuel, our bodies would convert up to 2.2 pounds of lean muscle mass a day, most of this energy going to the brain which is greedy in its energy needs.

Thankfully, the liver's ability to produce ketones enables your body to cut down on five times the protein it would otherwise need, as the liver will turn the fats from long-burning fuel that the brain is unable to use into a fast acting fuel that the brain can utilize without causing an excess of reactive oxygen species, the most dangerous form of oxidants. This process of turning fatty acids into fuel is known as ketogenesis and can fuel up to seventy-five percent of the brain's energy source requirements.

Using ketones for fuel as opposed to glucose is a powerful ability that not only helps our bodies in times of starvation, fasting, and dieting but also has a great many benefits for the brain's health.

Some of these benefits include:

- Ketones increase the number of mitochondrial cells and increase their effectiveness. This is important as mitochondrial cells are the type that can burn any of the body's fuel sources, thereby increasing the capacity of brain cells and protecting them from damage and neurodegenerative diseases in the process.

- Ketones are an efficient energy source. While glucose requires a large amount of oxygen to be utilized as fuel, ketones can be utilized at a much higher number with the same amount of oxygen. Not only does running more effectively give the brain more energy and clarity, but it also aids aging brain cells that lose their ability to effectively use glucose as fuel over time.

- Ketones protect the brain. It has been found that ketones act as a powerful antioxidant to rid the brain of damaging reactive oxygen species (ROS), the most dangerous form of oxidants. The oxidative stress that these ROSs cause has been found to be a crucial factor in the cause of many neurodegenerative diseases.

- Ketones balance glutamate and GABA. Glutamate is an important excitatory neurotransmitter and GABA is the brain's inhibitory neurotransmitter. While glutamate is essential for neural communication, regulation, learning, and memory formation, sometimes it can become a dangerous excitotoxin. Once glutamate becomes excitotoxic, it will damage and kill nerve cells, causing neurodegenerative conditions such as Parkinson's disease, multiple sclerosis, Lou Gehrig's disease, and Alzheimer's disease. Although it is still unclear as to how, it has been found that ketones can decrease the amount of excitotoxic glutamate, and increase the amount of GABA which prevents cell damage and improves brain function.

- Ketones trigger the brain-derived neurotrophic factor, also known as BDNF. While most of the neurons in the human brain are formed prenatally, certain areas of the brain retain the ability to produce new neurons from neural stem cells in a process known as neurogenesis. One of the most prominent proteins that stimulate and controls the neurogenesis process is BDNF.

This is important as it can encourage the growth and differentiation of new synapses and neurons. It can impact areas of the brain such as the hippocampus, basal forebrain, and cortex. These areas of the brain are vital to higher thinking, long-term memory, and learning. BDNF can also be present in the motor neurons, retina, prostate, saliva, and **kidneys.**

Whenever the body needs more energy, but there are not enough carbohydrates for fuel to meet its needs, the body will begin to increase ketone levels. If carbohydrates are restricted for a long length of time, such as for three or more days, then the ketone levels will begin to increase to an even higher level so that you are in a deep state of ketosis. These effects can have a profound effect on the human body, and they are experienced in the most healthy and safe way when following a controlled ketogenic diet. Despite this, most people never enter a deep ketosis state and therefore do not experience the numerous benefits it has to offer.

Ketones are created through the ketogenesis process when the liver converts fatty acids into the ketone body acetoacetate. This ketone can then be converted into two other types of ketones, beta-hydroxybutyrate, known as **BHB, and acetone.**

Acetone is a type of ketone that can sometimes be metabolized into glucose but is most often excreted as waste. Many people new to the ketogenic diet will complain of bad smelling breath with a weird fruity odor to it, which is a result of the acetone being expelled through the breath.

Over time your body will begin to create ketones more effectively and efficiently, meaning that if you test your ketone levels with urine strips, as is common, you may be concerned that your ketone levels drop. This happens because your body is no longer producing excess acetone, and is, in fact, a good sign. At this stage, once you have been keto-adapted for a few weeks, your body will begin to convert the acetoacetate into the more efficient ketone, BHB. This type of ketone is a better source of fuel, as it has undergone an additional chemical reaction in order to provide more energy than acetoacetate could alone. However, whether the ketone is BHB or acetoacetate, studies have shown that the body and brain prefer to use these ketones for energy, as they are used seventy percent more efficiently than glucose.

There is a three-stage process when it comes to your body creating ketones at the beginning of the diet or a fast.

Stage One: During this stage, which can last between six to twelve hours of fasting or being on the ketogenic diet, most of your body's energy is provided by glycogen. Hormone levels will shift, causing an increase in gluconeogenesis and the ability to burn your body's stored fats.

Stage Two: Within two to ten days of being on the ketogenic diet or fasting, your glycogen stores will be fully depleted, and gluconeogenesis will be providing the body with energy. At this stage, ketones are beginning to be produced, but only at low levels. You should have increased levels of acetone in your urine and blood and notice the well-known 'keto breath.'

This stage has a broad time-frame, as people can go into this stage at different speeds depending on their health and gender. Healthy men, overweight individuals, and those with insulin resistance tend to stay in phase two longer than healthy women.

Stage Three: After stage two, which could be anywhere from two to ten days, the ketogenic phase begins. Genetics, lifestyle factors, calorie count, carbohydrate level, and activity levels can all impact how quickly you enter stage three. This stage is characterized by the body's decrease in breaking down protein for energy and increase in turning fat into ketones for energy.

While you can experience ketosis both on the ketogenic diet and when fasting, it is much safer and healthier when on a controlled ketogenic diet. When in ketosis as results of fasting, the body has no food source and begins to convert lean muscle mass into glucose, thus resulting in rapid muscle loss. Going into ketosis through the ketogenic diet prevents this by giving your body all of the nutrients it needs.

You may lose weight more quickly when fasting, but this is a result of starvation and will leave you weak, depleted of nutrients, increases the chance of long-term negative health effects, and the rapid weight loss will leave your skin sagging.

No matter the reason you choose the ketogenic diet, you can experience reduced brain aging, prevent neurodegenerative diseases, boost brain function, decrease inflammation, improve brain cell growth and function, regulate neurotransmitters, and protect the brain from neuronal damage. Ketones are a wonderful option that will provide both brain and body with an efficient fuel source and health.

Chapter 2: The Health Benefits of Going Keto

You now know the history and the science behind the ketogenic diet, including how ketones are a better fuel for a healthy brain. Yet, there are still many health benefits of the ketogenic diet, and in this chapter, we will introduce them to you.

Weight Loss

Losing weight can give you more energy and make you feel better about yourself. While there is nothing wrong with being fat, and parts of society are slowly learning to stop fat shaming, it is true that being at a lower body weight increases the chance of better health.

While many diets can help you lose weight, the

ketogenic diet is unique. On typical diets, which are higher in carbohydrates, your body will develop a blood sugar crash whenever you run out of glucose to use for fuel. Despite having the ability to use fat as fuel, the body is not adjusted to doing so. Yet, on the ketogenic diet, you are providing your body with long-lasting fuel which does not cause blood sugar crashes, leaving you feeling satisfied and full throughout the day. Thus, you are able to eat fewer calories without feeling deprived or the need to overeat to compensate, helping you to lose weight.

Another way in which the ketogenic diet promotes better weight loss is by burning off your body's stores of adipose. As your body is constantly burning fat and ketones as fuel, it gains the ability to easily and seamlessly burn off your body fat.

Anti-Aging

The mitochondrial cells are imperative for our survival. These cells produce ninety percent of the energy the human body requires. However, it has been found that occasionally during the process of creating energy, electrons will escape and cause a reaction with oxygen molecules, forming free radicals such as peroxide and superoxide.

These free radicals wreak havoc on our cells and are known as reactive oxygen species. Thankfully, we do not have to accept these as a part of life. Antioxidants are able to help clean up these oxidants, thus protecting our cells. Mitochondrial cells contain a high level of such antioxidants, but with age the antioxidant properties of these cells decrease, leading to higher numbers of oxidants.

If we want to protect our health and live longer we need to look after our mitochondrial cells, and one of the most powerful ways in which to do this is through the ketogenic diet. Not only has the process of ketosis been found to increase the overall number of mitochondrial cells, but it has also been found to increase antioxidant levels, and reduce reactive oxygen species.

Parkinson's Disease

Parkinson's is a degenerative nervous system disease that can cause symptoms such as tremors, rigidity, fatigue, cognitive impairment, depression, pain, slurred speech, and movement difficulties. The exact cause of Parkinson's disease is still yet unknown, but it has been found that mitochondria cell dysfunction does play an intricate role.

Most of the symptoms caused by Parkinson's disease appear to be caused by oxidative stress damage and cell death as a result of this mitochondrial cell dysfunction. More specifically, this damage causes deterioration of the dopamine-producing cells in the brain, and as they continue to deteriorate, the symptoms progress. While not every patient's symptoms are the same, the one consistency is that the available drugs for Parkinson's disease have a multitude of undesirable side effects and over time become less effective in managing the symptoms.

With the ketogenic diet's powerful ability to multiply and heal the mitochondria and increase antioxidants, it has been found to help ease the symptoms and delay the progression of this debilitating disease.

Epilepsy

The ketogenic diet obviously has a wonderful healing ability for patients with epilepsy. Despite the invention of anticonvulsant drugs during the 1900s, the ketogenic diet has remained a viable standard in treatment for nearly a century.

Between the years of 2001 to 2006, Dr. Susan Masino from Trinity College conducted a controlled randomized study of 145 children on the ketogenic diet. These children experienced daily seizures and had previously experienced no success on at least two types of anticonvulsant drugs. The children placed on the ketogenic diet experienced a significant decrease in seizure activity, where thirty-eight percent of the children had a fifty percent or more reduction in seizure activity. Seven percent of the children experienced a reduction of over ninety percent.

Another study done between the years of 1995 and 2001 found that the ketogenic diet was safe for epileptic patients and that any experienced side effects were during the early process of ketosis, easily managed, and short-lived.

Alzheimer's Disease

Alzheimer's disease is the sixth leading cause of death in America, and between the years 2000 and 2015, deaths from Alzheimer's disease have increased by a startling one-hundred-twenty-three percent. There is neither a known cause nor treatment of Alzheimer's disease at this time. Yet, scientists do know many of the contributing factors of the disease and are constantly coming closer to finding answers in the treatment of this devastating condition.

Some of the known contributing factors for Alzheimer's include a variation in the APOE protein gene, mitochondrial dysfunction, degeneration of brain cells, immune system dysfunction, repeated head injuries, and malnutrition. Each of these factors can cause a build-up of plaque and neurofibrillary tangles in the brain, resulting in chronic inflammation, oxidative stress, and mitochondrial dysfunction. It is a vicious cycle where one factor worsens another, causing the disease to progress further.

One of the effects of Alzheimer's disease is insulin resistance of the neurons in the brain. This makes it difficult for the cells to absorb glucose, which slowly starves them of fuel. The ketogenic diet has been found to be an effective treatment of insulin resistance, as ketones provide the brain with a fuel source, along with helping them better absorb glucose through the gluconeogenesis process. Some of the other benefits the ketogenic diet has on Alzheimer's is a decrease in oxidative stress, an increase in mitochondrial production, neuron cell protection from antioxidants, regulation of the glutamatergic system, promotes the expression of BDNF, decreases blood sugar levels, and activates the cellular cleaning process of autophagy.

Numerous studies have shown significant improvement of Alzheimer's patients on the ketogenic diet, and it has been found that a single high-carbohydrate meal can backtrack the benefits experienced.

Diabetes

Whenever making dietary changes as a diabetic, it is important to consult with your doctor and closely track all of your vitals and levels to ensure your safety.

There have been many tests conducted on the safety and effectiveness of the ketogenic diet for type II diabetes. One such study led by Dr. Eric Westman of Duke University compared a traditional ketogenic diet to a low-calorie diet. This study showed that the ketogenic group experienced an increase in weight loss, a reduction in glycated hemoglobin, and many of the patients were able to either decrease or discontinue their diabetic medications.

Another such study comparing the ketogenic

diet to both reduced-calorie diets and low-glycemic diets found that the patients who were obese and had type II diabetes experienced superior results on every criterion compared to the patients on the other diets. These patients experienced a greater decrease in hemoglobin A1C, increased HDL cholesterol, decreased LDL cholesterol, increased weight loss, and a greater reduction in diabetic medications.

Studies regarding type I diabetes with the ketogenic diet are seriously limited. For this reason, it cannot definitively be stated whether or not it is safe for those with type I diabetes. But, that does not mean there are no studies whatsoever.

In one study a young girl with epilepsy and type I diabetes was placed on a standard ketogenic diet for a period of fifteen months. Once the study began the girl experienced exceptional improvement in seizure activity,

A1C levels, and glycemic control, all without any significant side effects.

In another study, a nineteen-year-old male with type I diabetes was put on a modified ketogenic diet for nearly seven months. During the study, he was able to discontinue his insulin medication and his pancreas restored some of its ability to naturally produce insulin.

More studies on the ketogenic diet and type I diabetes are greatly needed, but it is clear from the evidence that ketosis could be a powerful and viable treatment option.

High-Cholesterol

High levels of LDL and VLDL cholesterol are a serious problem that continues to rise. You may be concerned that the ketogenic diet could raise your cholesterol; after all, fats supposedly raise cholesterol levels. While this is true, it is not the complete story.

Unhealthy fats, such as vegetable fats, can raise bad cholesterol, the LDL and VLDL. Healthy fats that you will be eating on the ketogenic diet, on the other hand, raise good cholesterol which in turns lowers bad cholesterol. Put simply, the ketogenic diet and many of the foods you can enjoy on it have been proven to improve cholesterol levels.

In one long-term study, sixty-six obese patients with high cholesterol participated in the ketogenic diet. The results were encouraging. The patients not only raised their good cholesterol, HDL, they also lowered the overall levels of LDL cholesterol, blood glucose, and triglycerides. While on the ketogenic diet they also lost a significant portion of the weight.

Polycystic Ovary Syndrome (PCOS)

PCOS is the most common endocrine disorder affecting women. This condition causes insulin resistance, obesity, body hair growth, hyperinsulinemia, abnormal menstruation, fatigue, infertility, and more. While the cause of PCOS is still unknown, genetics, inflammation, excessive insulin, and excessive androgen may play a role.

The ketogenic diet has successfully improved insulin, testosterone, body weight, and infertility in women placed on a twenty-four-week ketogenic study. Another study found that reducing carbohydrates improved hormone imbalances, ovulation, insulin, and fertility.

In one study on the mental health of women diagnosed with PCOS, it was found that a high-protein and low-carbohydrate diet was able to significantly improve their mental health, unlike the control group, which had no change.

Multiple studies have shown that women with PCOS who had previously been unable to become pregnant became fertile again after a few short weeks on the ketogenic diet, making it a promising treatment option.

Decreased Inflammation

A wide variety of chronic diseases cause increased pain and inflammation. However, the ketogenic diet has been shown to greatly reduce this inflammation, which therefore helps the pain levels and other symptoms the diseases may cause.

Non-Alcoholic Fatty Liver Disease

People with non-alcoholic fatty liver diseases are predisposed to fat collecting in the liver. While there is a large portion of obese patients with the fatty liver disease, it can manifest itself in people who are only slightly overweight or even at a healthy weight. The number of people with this disease has been greatly increased and with that the number of needed liver transplants. Increasing the available treatment options is vital.

The ketogenic diet has been found to be a viable treatment option for non-alcoholic fatty liver disease in a large number of cases. In one pilot study, five patients followed the ketogenic diet for six months, and afterward, four of the five patients showed significant weight loss and improvements in fibrosis, steatosis, and inflammation.

Cancer

The ketogenic diet has become increasingly more popular not just for cancer prevention, but in cancer treatment, as well. This is because while most of the cells in your body can convert to using ketones as fuel, cancer and tumor cells are only able to use glucose for fuel. Going on a low-carbohydrate diet essentially starves the cancer cells for fuel, often either halting or reversing their growth within a matter of days.

In one study, nine patients with rapid disease progression that had been unresponsive to any cancer treatment were placed on the ketogenic diet for a period of twenty-six to twenty-eight days. Five of the patients experienced either partial remission or stability.

Multiple Sclerosis

Multiple sclerosis is a debilitating and degenerative disease that causes mass nerve damage, affecting the communication between the brain and body in the process. Multiple sclerosis, also known as MS, often effects movement, vision, balance, memory, and more.

In one randomized controlled study of forty-eight people with MS, some participants were placed on the ketogenic diet while others were placed on scheduled fasting. The results revealed that both fasting and the ketogenic diet greatly improved the patients' conditions and that combining intermittent fasting with the ketogenic diet may be even more powerful.

The way in which the ketogenic diet protects and repairs brain cells, reduces inflammation, and increases memory could prove to be a powerful treatment option in this devastating disease.

Mood Stabilization

One in five Americans has a mental illness, which are over forty-million people. Thankfully, the ketogenic diet has been found to have a mood stabilizing effect on a wide range of mental illnesses, including depression, anxiety, and bipolar disorder.

While studies on human participants are limited, there is a great deal of research showing that a ketogenic diet is an effective option for mental health. One study on two women with type II bipolar disorder found that both women experienced a mood stabilizing effect that was more effective than medication. The women were on the diet for a period of two and three years, and both tolerated it well.

There are many studies showing rats and mice reacting well to a ketogenic diet. In one such study, it was found that the ketogenic diet was just as effective in rats as antidepressants. The rats spent more time active and did not show any behavioral despair.

Appetite Control

When eating a standard diet, your blood sugar is constantly going up and down throughout the day. Not only does this affect your energy levels through both highs and lows, but it also controls your hunger. Whether or not your body needs more fuel, when your blood sugar drops it will tell you that you are hungry, causing you to overeat.

Since your blood sugar stays stable and you have a long-burning fuel source on the ketogenic diet you are able to go longer periods without eating.

There are many health benefits to the ketogenic diet, which are even more pronounced when paired with intermittent fasting. While the ketogenic diet may be a lifestyle change, it can be easily managed and well worth the change.

Chapter 3:
The Fundamentals of the Ketogenic Diet

At its core, the ketogenic diet is a low-carbohydrate, moderate-protein, and high-fat diet. Yet, knowing this does not help you know how to actually follow the diet plan. In this chapter, we will discuss how to follow the various types of ketogenic diets and how to tailor it to your needs.

The Standard Ketogenic Diet

This is the version of the ketogenic diet that most people utilize, as it is versatile and meets the needed nutritional levels for most people. On this version, fats should make up seventy to eighty percent of your daily calorie intake, protein should make up twenty to twenty-five percent, and carbohydrates should only make up five to ten percent.

While some people believe you should eat a lower protein diet, their cause for that has been debunked. They believe that eating excess protein will kick your body out of ketosis, due to the gluconeogenesis process. This process transmutes lactate, glycerol, and amino acids into glucose for the few cells that are unable to survive off of ketones and fat. However, the gluconeogenesis process is very stable, and it will not increase the production of glucose based on how many proteins you eat.

Many people do not eat enough protein on the ketogenic diet due to fear of the gluconeogenesis process, but this fear causes many people to lose muscle tone as if you do not eat enough protein the gluconeogenesis will begin converting your lean muscle mass into glucose.

Eating the correct proportion of macronutrients, those being carbohydrates, fats, and proteins is extremely important. Thankfully, there are many free-to-use ketogenic macro calculators online that make eating the correct proportions of each food source easy.

You can lose, maintain, or gain weight on the ketogenic diet, depending on your goals and your doctor's recommendations. To do this, simply put your weight, activity level, and weight goals into a ketogenic macro calculator. You can easily reach your goals simply by eating the recommended amount of calories a day.

The Targeted Ketogenic Diet

While the standard ketogenic diet is effective for a large percentage of people, those who lead a more active lifestyle may need to try one of the variant options. The most simple and all-purpose variation is the targeted ketogenic diet. On this version, you simply eat a small serving of a high-carbohydrate food, such as a sweet potato or fruit, thirty-minutes before exercising. This is done because while cardio and flexibility exercise can be performed completely on the ketogenic diet, high-intensity exercises such as bodybuilding and high-intensity interval training, known as HIIT, require glucose for fuel.

This is due to how our muscles process energy. Any exercise that lasts less than ten seconds will use ATP and creatine phosphate that is stored in the muscles for immediate use. This energy source is used whenever someone goes all-out in using their muscles in a limited span of time, for instance, when you begin to race someone at full-speed.

High-intensity exercises, such as bodybuilding and HIIT that last somewhere between ten seconds and two minutes rely on glucose for fuel. If you are on a standard ketogenic diet then these muscles will be lacking in fuel, making your strength and stamina decrease.

The targeted ketogenic diet solves this problem by having you consume enough carbohydrates in order to fuel a workout, about twenty-five to fifty grams worth, but a small enough serving so that you can ensure you burn off all of the glucose and maintain a state of ketosis.

The Cyclical Ketogenic Diet

The cyclical ketogenic diet, like the targeted version, is for highly active individuals. Unlike the targeted ketogenic diet, the cyclical version is only for advanced bodybuilders or HIIT trainers; as you follow the cyclical ketogenic diet while only being at an intermediate level, you will be unable to maintain ketosis.

On the cyclical ketogenic diet, you will eat five

to six days of the standard ketogenic diet, with two high-carbohydrate days. The purpose of this is to completely fill up your body's glucose and glycogen stores, which you will then burn through the following week. The purpose is to burn through this stored glucose and glycogen quickly as to re-enter ketosis, so in order to successfully follow the ketogenic diet you need to be not only at an advanced level of your desired high-intensity exercise, but you also need to follow a strict workout routine.

The High-Protein Ketogenic Diet

This version of the diet can be combined with either the standard, targeted, or cyclical versions. The purpose of the high-protein ketogenic diet is to boost protein levels for bodybuilders or for people who have health conditions that improve with increased protein levels.

The high-protein ketogenic diet simply

consumes between 1 gram of protein and 1.3 grams of protein per pound of body weight. This protein can come from a variety of sources, and it is good to mix it up in order to receive the best nutrition possible. Protein from eggs, beef, chicken, shrimp, nuts, fish, dairy, lamb, and organ meats, are all good options.

Reaching Ketosis

The most difficult part of the ketogenic diet is the beginning, while your body tries to adjust from running off of carbohydrates into becoming keto-adapted. This process leads to what is known as the 'keto flu', where your body is going through a period of shock and withdrawals, which can cause symptoms such as headaches, nausea, irritability, muscle aches, dizziness, difficulties concentrating, stomach pains, and sugar cravings. This keto flu typically lasts about a week, although some people may experience it for up to two weeks.

In order to experience as smooth of a transition as possible, it is important to follow a few steps.

Stay Hydrated

It is extremely important to focus on hydration when starting out on the ketogenic diet, as many people end up dehydrated which not only worsens symptoms such as headaches and dizziness, it also becomes dangerous. This happens because when you reduce your carbohydrate intake the levels of glycogen in your body plummet, and since glycogen cells bond to cells of water, it will cause large portions of water to be flushed from the body. This can be worsened if the keto flu is causing you to experience diarrhea.

It is commonly recommended to consume one ounce per pound of body weight each day. If you weigh 160 pounds then you should be drinking 80 ounces of water a day. Be sure to never drink more than a liter in the span of an hour, or else your liver will be unable to process all of the newly introduced fluid.

Refuel on Electrolytes

When the body dumps large portions of water electrolytes go with it, and it is important to refuel the electrolytes right along with the water. One easy way to do this is by drinking ketogenic electrolyte drinks. You can also achieve the same effect by consuming sodium, potassium, and magnesium through your diet and supplements.

To ensure you are getting enough sodium, try to consume between four to six grams of a mineral-rich salt, such as pink Himalayan sea salt, each day.

Potassium is highly concentrated in many foods, such as avocados and wild caught salmon, so as long as you eat a nutritionally balanced version of the ketogenic diet you should be able to easily maintain high enough levels. Try to aim for about four grams of potassium a day.

It is recommended to consume 400 milligrams of magnesium a day, and you are able to get nearly half of that from one hundred grams of almonds. One hundred milligrams of spinach contains seventy-nine grams. If you are having difficulty getting enough magnesium in your diet, supplements are readily available and inexpensive.

Eat as Needed

You may want to start losing weight and seeing the results of your hard work right away, but be careful to eat enough during the beginning. Since your body is not yet used to using fat as the fuel you may feel hungry more often, which could lead to weakness, stress, and overeating later on if you do not feed your body as needed. You don't have to eat a large meal every time you are hungry, but just allowing yourself to eat a small snack can help increase energy and reduce cravings.

Light Exercise

Strenuous exercises such as weightlifting or marathons should be avoided in the beginning. While your body is still adjusting to its new way of eating, you will have less stamina and energy, making any strenuous exercise much more taxing on the body and will cause it to worsen the keto flu symptoms. On the other hand, light exercises such as yoga and walking may help decrease the symptoms and improve energy levels.

Sleep Well

When the body is unable to get adequate levels of sleep levels of the stress hormone will increase and leptin, an important hormone to hell signal to your brain that you are full and no longer need to eat, will decrease. Not only do both of these hormones being out of sync can cause weight loss difficulties, but it will also make you more stressed and increase the intensity of your other symptoms from the keto flu.

If you are having a difficult time falling or to stay asleep, try meditating, turning off electronics an hour before bed, soaking in a hot bath, or taking a magnesium supplement before bed.

If you are able to successfully maintain these points, then you will find your flu symptoms greatly decrease and before long you will begin to feel better.

Chapter 4: What You Can and Cannot Eat

While the main principle of the ketogenic diet is eating the correct proportion of fats, carbohydrates, and proteins, it is important to eat these from healthy sources. Otherwise, you may develop nutritional deficiencies and miss out on many of the beneficial effects of this lifestyle.

In this chapter, we will explore some of the food options you have on the ketogenic diet to get you well on your way to success. Not only will you learn what you can eat, but you will learn why it is good for you, as well. Weight loss and health do not have to mean eating tasteless food.

Avocados

Avocados are a wonderful choice on the ketogenic diet, as they only contain 4 net carbohydrates. They are also a good source of healthy fat, containing 29 grams per avocado. This fruit is a good source of potassium, which is an important electrolyte for maintaining cellular and electrical function. One avocado contains 975 milligrams of potassium. Avocados are also high in vitamins K, C, B5, B6, E, and folate.

Avocados are high in oleic acid, which is the type of fat that is responsible for olive oil's heart-healthy benefits, has been shown to reduce inflammation, and has a beneficial effect on genes that are linked to cancer. The fats in Avocado oil have been shown to be resistant to heat-induced oxidation, making them a safer cooking option. They are high in soluble fiber, which improves gut health and digestion. Avocados can also help lower cholesterol, increase nutrient absorption, increase antioxidants, and more.

Olives

Olives are a stone fruit which contains a high level of the healthy fat, oleic acid. They also contain high levels of vitamin E, iron, copper, calcium, sodium, and the antioxidants oleuropein, hydroxytyrosol tyrosol, oleanolic acid, and quercetin. The high antioxidant properties help fight against cancer, heart disease, inflammation and fight off infection.

While high blood pressure and high cholesterol lead to heart disease, olives have been shown to reduce these to healthy levels. Olives also can help prevent bone loss and improve blood circulation, blood sugar, and brain health.

Sardines

Sardines are a scary food to many as they are smelly and often contain skin and bones. But, they are an incredibly nutritious food when packed in olive oil, and can be bought as fillets with the bones removed. There are also many recipes that make them incredibly tasty. Sardines contain high levels of omega-3, which lowers cholesterol, supports heart health and boosts brain health. Selenium is an important mineral for thyroid and adrenal health, which many people do not eat enough of. Many people are deficient in vitamin D, and very few people have optimal levels, thankfully, sardines are high in this very important vitamin.

Coconut Oil

Whereas most fats are long-chain triglycerides, many of the fats in coconut oil are medium-chain triglycerides. This means that they are able to go straight to the liver and be processed as fuel, giving you a quick burst of energy. Some people may worry about the high level of saturated fat in coconut oil, however, the saturated fats in coconut are healthy and have been proven to help lower LDL cholesterol and raise HDL cholesterol. The high density of MCTs in coconut oil can help you burn off fat more quickly and efficiently. Coconut oil even kills harmful pathogens such as viruses, bacteria, and fungi.

Coconut oil is known to reduce hunger, increase ketones, increase skin and hair health, boosts brain function, prevents yeast infections, and more!

Walnuts

Walnuts are a wonderful source of fat, fiber, antioxidants, vitamins, and minerals. The high antioxidant levels of walnuts prevent oxidative damage, including oxidative damage caused by LDL cholesterol. Walnuts are also high in omega-3, decrease inflammation, improve gut health, may reduce the risk of cancer, aids weight loss and appetite control, controls blood sugar, lowers high blood pressure, improves male fertility, supports brain health, and they are easily added into the diet.

Almonds

Almonds have now long been known as a health food, yet many people are still ignorant of the amazing benefits they have to offer. Almonds are not only tasty and satisfying, they are also lower LDL cholesterol while raising HDL cholesterol, are high in antioxidants, are high in fiber and help prevent colon cancer, reduce the risk of heart disease and heart attack, control blood sugar, lower blood pressure, aid weight loss, boost brain health, improves bone strength and durability, reduces inflammation, increases energy, and the list goes on!

Pecans

Pecans are not just delicious; they are high in zinc and antioxidants, which are crucial for a healthy immune system. Pecans have high levels of flavonoids, which aid in weight maintenance and help prevent chronic disease. The high levels of beta-carotene and vitamin E help reduce chronic inflammation. Pecans also lower cholesterol, improve blood sugar, boost the brain, protect important cells in your organs, reduces stress from free radicals, prevents osteoporosis, and more!

Grass-Fed Butter

Butter has been vilified greatly in the past, but despite the low-fat craze of the late 90s and early 2000s, grass-fed butter has many health benefits. You may not think there is a difference in the butter you can find in the dairy department, but, grass-fed butter is much higher in nutrients and health benefits. For instance, grass-fed butter is five times higher in the conjugated linoleic fatty acid, which reduces body fat, lessens the risk of cancer and cardiovascular disease, modulates the immune system, reduces inflammation, and improves bone mass. Studies show that people who eat grass-fed butter greatly reduce the risk of heart disease. It is a high source of vitamin A, boosts energy, suppresses appetite, and protects eye health.

Broccoli

Broccoli is a wonderful choice, not just because it is low in net carbohydrates, but because it is amazingly healthy. Broccoli contains high levels of fiber, vitamin A, beta-carotene, thiamine, riboflavin, niacin, vitamins B6, C, E, B1, B9, K, manganese, omega-3, flavonoids, antioxidants, and the list just goes on! There is a reason your mother always told you to eat your broccoli.

Some of the amazing health benefits broccoli has is aiding in digestion, boosts liver health and function, improves memory and cognition, keeps hair healthy, reduces allergies, anti-inflammatory, controls blood sugar, improves metabolism, improves eye health, prevents heart disease, and more.

Asparagus

Asparagus is high in insoluble fiber which helps in keeping you feel full, satisfied, and lose weight. It also helps reduce cholesterol and aid in constipation. High levels of the amino acid asparagine help flush excess fluid, reducing the likelihood of UTIs in the process, Asparagus, especially purple asparagus, is full of anthocyanins, which is what gives many vegetables and fruits their purple, blue, and red hues. This antioxidant helps reduce free radical damage. Asparagus also reduces bloating, improves gut health, improves mental health, and is high in B vitamins, vitamin E, vitamin K, and folic acid.

Zucchini

Zucchini is a great nutrient-dense food that is

high in fiber, vitamin B6, riboflavin, potassium, manganese, folate, vitamin C, vitamin K, antioxidants, and phytonutrients. It is also a wonderful option to turn into vegetable noodles for a low-carbohydrate option.

Zucchini also helps aid in digestion, reduces inflammation, slows down aging from free radicals, lowers blood sugar, improves eye health, reduces fatigue, boosts the mood, improves adrenal and thyroid function, aids in weight loss, and increases collagen formation.

Mushrooms

Mushrooms are extremely healthy, so much so that they have been used in medicine throughout Asia since ancient times. Mushrooms are high in antioxidants which protect you from disease, boost the immune system, and prevent cell damage from free radicals. They are high in beta-glucan, a type of soluble fiber that improves cholesterol and heart health. Mushrooms are high in B vitamins such as riboflavin, niacin, and pantothenic acid which help with red blood cell health, the digestive system, healthy skin, the nervous system, and hormonal balance. They are high in copper, which is essential for healthy red blood cells, and maintaining healthy bones and nerves. Mushrooms also help prevent cancer, treat anemia, improve nutrient absorption, improve weight loss, lower blood pressure, and more.

Green Beans

While most beans are not allowed on the ketogenic diet, green beans are low in carbohydrates and high in fiber, making them a very healthy keto options. Green beans are high in vitamins A, C, B6, K, and folic acid, as well as calcium, iron, silicon, manganese, potassium, and copper. The high flavonoid content they offer lowers the risk of heart disease. They reduce cancer risks, especially colon cancer. Green beans also lower blood sugar, boosts the immune system, improves eye health, strengthens bones, improve gastrointestinal conditions, and are great for prenatal care.

Blackberries

One of the few fruits allowed on the ketogenic diet, blackberries are full of disease-fighting antioxidants such as flavonoids, phenolic acids, flavonols, and anthocyanosides. This powerful berry fights and prevents cancer, protects vascular function, boosts mood and cognitive function, improves digestion, lowers cholesterol and improves heart health, boosts the immune system, increases bone health, aids in skin health, improves eye health, and normalizes blood clotting.

Strawberries

Strawberries are not just a delicious fruit; they are low in carbohydrates and packed with important vitamins and minerals such as vitamins C and K, folate, manganese, potassium, magnesium, and antioxidants. Strawberries are high in flavonoids that help boost cardiovascular health and improve blood flow. They are high in iodine, vitamin C, and phytochemicals, which improve the nervous system and boosts brain health. The antioxidants are a wonderful cancer preventative and prevent strokes. Strawberries are also great for skin health, reduce aging, boosts collagen, improves eye health, lowers high blood pressure, improves glycemic index control, boosts the immune system, lowers inflammation, aids in weight loss, strengthens bone density, and reduces constipation.

Raspberries

Raspberries are not just delicious and healthy, they aid in weight loss thanks to their high concentration of fiber and manganese. Their ellagic acid is a phenolic compound which can help prevent and stop the growth of cancer. Raspberries help keep skin youthful by reducing age spots and wrinkles and protecting it from the sun. They also help aid in eye health, prevent infections, strengthen the immune system, improve mental health, and reduce inflammation.

Shrimp

Shrimp, also known as prawns, is full of important vitamins and minerals including vitamins A, D, E, B6, and B12, iron, calcium, sodium, zinc, phosphorus, magnesium, potassium, iodine, thiamine, riboflavin, and niacin. Shrimp aids in weight loss, increases leptin levels, improves skin health, relieves eyestrain, reduces hair loss, increases cardiovascular health and reduces blood clots, increases bone strength and density, improves brain health, lowers the risks of cancer, decreases menstrual pain, increases red blood cell count, and improves thyroid function.

Grass-Fed Beef

While red meats are often vilified, grass-fed beef is in fact very healthy with many health benefits. Like grass-fed butter, grass-fed beef contains high levels of conjugated linoleic acid or CLA. This antioxidant protects against heart disease, diabetes, cancer, and promotes weight loss. Grass-fed beef also has two to four times the amount of omega-3 as its grain-fed counterpart. Beef is high in niacin, vitamin B6, selenium, zinc, phosphorus, B12, iron, potassium, magnesium, copper, thiamin, and folate.

Liver

While organ meats have fallen out of favor in modern western society, they are full of vitamins and minerals, especially the liver. The liver is high in vitamins A, B12, B6, C, D, potassium, choline, iron, phosphorus, zinc, copper, thiamin, riboflavin, folate, biotin, the list goes on. The liver is essentially one of the best natural multivitamins.

Many people worry about eating liver because it is compared to a sieve that catches all of the harmful chemicals in the body. But, this comparison is not quite accurate. The liver does remove harmful toxins from the body, but it does not hold onto them, it expels them. Of course, it is best to get grass-fed organic liver if possible, but there is no need to worry about the liver being any higher in toxins than any other meat.

Chapter 5: The History and Science Behind Intermittent Fasting

Fasting has been a part of all of human history, whether, for health, religion, ethics, or rituals, fasting have remained a large part of many cultures. There is a reason why it has been held in such high regard and has remained a part of many societies. In this chapter, we will go over the history and the science behind fasting, letting you better understand how it can help you in the process.

The History

Fasting was commonly used therapeutically in ancient Greece. The physician Hippocrates would recommend fasting for patients with certain symptoms, especially those who had lost their appetite. Some physicians believed that if you lost your appetite it could be detrimental to eat, as fasting was thought to be a natural part of the healing process.

Fasting is an integral part of many religions. Buddhist monks and nuns frequently do not eat after the noon meal each day, following the Vinaya Pitaka. They consider fasting in this way good for health and a disciplined regime to aid in meditation. Many Buddhists will also practice fasting during times of intense meditation and study. During this time they completely avoid animal products aside from milk, processed foods, and the five pungent foods, which are garlic, welsh onion, asana, garlic chives, and leeks.

Many Christian denominations practice fasting; both during specific seasons and as individuals as they feel led by the Holy Spirit. In Western Christianity, some of the denominations that practice fasting are the

Catholic Church, Methodist Church, Reformed Church, and the Anglican Church. The most prominent time to fast is during Lent, which is a forty-day partial fast commemorating when Christ was tempted in the desert. While some denominations observe the full forty-day fast, others choose to primarily fast on Ash Wednesday and Good Friday.

Fasting is a part of the Hindu religion. There is not one type or method of fasting, as it differs greatly based on the person's individual beliefs and local customs. Some people will fast by not partaking of any food or water from the previous day's sunset until forty-eight minutes after the following day's sunrise. Some limit themselves to a single meal during the day, or others choose to obtain from certain types of food. Some are of the times in which Hindus will fast include specific days of the month, such as Ekadashi, Pradosham, and Purnima. Fasting on Tuesdays is common in both southern and northwestern India. Thursday fasting is common in northern India. Fasting during religious festivals is also common.

In Muslim culture it is believed that fasting is more than just abstaining from food or drink, it is also about abstaining from immoral behavior. Fasting is used to strengthen control of impulses and to help the person develop better behavior. During the sacred month of Ramadan people strive to purify both body and soul to increase their good deeds and God-consciousness. Muslims try to improve their body and health by reducing food intake, and overindulgence is greatly discouraged.

Jews traditionally fast six days of the year, and with the exception of Yom Kippur, fasting is never permitted on Shabbat. For Yom Kippur, every man or woman above the age of bar mitzvah or bat mitzvah is expected to fast, unless it would put their health in critical danger. For the Jews, it means completely abstaining from all food and drink, even water.

Hunger strikes, a form of fasting, have been a form of peaceful protests for centuries. In pre-Christian Ireland, a hunger strike was known as Cealachan or Troscadh, and it had specific rules and civic codes. The fast would be held at the front door of the home of the offender. Many scholars speculate this is because the culture placed high importance on hospitality, and allowing a person to die at your doorstep would be a great dishonor. Others claim that there is no evidence showing that the fast may be until death and that the fast would last one full night. While the exact reason is unknown, it is known that these fasting would often be undertaken in order to recover debts or justice for other wrongs. There are even legends of St. Patrick using hunger strikes.

Prior to 1861, a similar type of hunger protest was practiced in India, and in their culture, it would also be held at the front door of someone who had wronged them, such as a debtor. While no longer practiced in India, this is an ancient form of protest that goes back to around the time of four hundred to seven hundred BC. This is known, as it appears in the Ramayana, which was composed around that time.

During the early 20th century, suffragettes often underwent hunger strikes in British prisons. The first was Marion Dunlop, but she was released because the police did not want to turn her into a martyr. Many other suffragettes also used hunger strikes to further their cause, but British authorities would subject them to force-feeding, which was often categorized as a form of torture by the women. Mary Clarke, sister of Emmeline Pankhurst, even died after being force-fed and many other women developed serious health problems as a result.

During 1952, an Indian revolutionary, Potti Sriramulu, died after undertaking a fifty eight-day hunger strike. He fought in order to achieve the formation of a separate state after the Indian independence and to be known as Andhra State. Potti Sriramulu's sacrifice was instrumental to the State's Reorganization Commission, and he is now revered as Amarajeevi or Immortal Being.

There have been a number of notable hunger strikes in Cuba. One such example is of Guillermo Fariñas, who completed a seven-month hunger strike in order to protest the internet censorship by the Cuban government. Fariñas ended his hunger strike in autumn of 2006, once he developed severe health problems. He was soon thereafter awarded with a Cyber-Freedom prize by Reporters Without Borders.

The Science

In this portion, we will go over the health benefits of intermittent fasting. Unlike long fasting cleanses that may take up to two weeks, intermittent fasting is done for shorter periods, most often for several hours, but sometimes up to a few days. Studies are increasingly showing not only the powerful weight loss abilities from intermittent fasting but the beneficial effects on health, as well.

The human body processes fasting in the same way as it does the ketogenic diet. Not only does this mean that the two work well hand in hand, but it means that if you are on the ketogenic diet then intermittent fasting will be more natural and easier to manage. With both intermittent fasting and with the ketogenic diet, your body will begin by burning through all of the glycogen stores in your muscles and liver. This state typically takes between six to twenty-four hours, but it can take up to a week for people with diabetes. Once your body burns through the glycogen stores, it will begin to convert protein and lean muscle mass into glucose with the gluconeogenesis process. Not much longer after that your body will finally start producing ketones to use as a fuel source, which has many health benefits.

Increased Growth Hormone

The human growth hormone, produced in the pituitary gland, is important. This hormone is responsible for cell growth and regeneration, increasing muscle mass, maintaining brain and tissue health, and bone density.

The human growth hormone skyrockets during times of fasting, studies show that it can rise up to five times its normal level. This is important, as the growth hormone reduces as we age and lower levels are attributed to a decrease in lean muscle mass, increased adipose tissue, and the thinning of the skin. Studies have shown that increased levels of the human growth hormone, also known as HGH, increase total fat loss, abdominal fat loss, muscle strength and tone, bone health, and improve cardiovascular health.

Weight Loss

Rather than burning off the calories from the meals you have eaten on any given day, intermittent fasting gives your body the time to burn off fat, instead.

While the increase in the human growth hormone does help aid in weight loss, a large portion of why intermittent fasting helps with weight loss is due to the restriction of calories. A study in 2014 found that fasting leads to significant weight loss, and over a period of three to twenty-four weeks was able to decrease body weight by a total of three to eight percent.

Less Muscle Loss

Dieting by restricting calories typically leads to a loss of lean muscle mass. However, a 2011 study found that while calorie restriction and intermittent fasting may both lead to similar fat loss results, intermittent fasting led to less muscle loss than calorie restriction.

Decreases Insulin Resistance

Studies have found that intermittent fasting is as effective in reducing insulin resistance as calorie restriction. Another study found that intermittent fasting significantly reduced blood sugar levels. Not only does reducing insulin resistance lessen your chance of diabetes, or improve diabetes if you already have it, it also helps your body transport glucose more effectively, and prevents blood sugar spikes and crashes.

Reduces Inflammation

Inflammation is a normal part of the immune system, yet chronically increased levels of inflammation have been shown to lead to chronic conditions such as heart disease, rheumatoid arthritis, and cancer. Studies have shown that intermittent fasting for one month leads to significant decreases in inflammation levels, and another study found the same effect when people fasted for twelve hours a day for a month.

Improved Heart Health

One of the leading causes of death around the world is heart disease. It is estimated that this condition causes 31.5% of deaths globally. One of the most effective ways to minimize your risk of heart disease is to improve your diet and lifestyle, and studies have shown that adding intermittent fasting into your routine may help.

In one study it was found that adding alternate-day fasting in for eight weeks was able to decrease LDL, the bad, cholesterol by twenty-five percent and blood triglycerides by thirty-two percent. Another study of over one-hundred obese adults revealed that fasting for three weeks was able to significantly decrease blood pressure, blood triglycerides, total cholesterol, and LDL cholesterol.

Boosts Brain Function

While most of the studies on brain function and fasting are on animals, and more human studies are needed, the results are promising. One study in mice found that intermittent fasting for eleven months improved both brain function and structure. Another study found that fasting may improve overall brain health, as well as increasing the generation of nerve cells, and enhancing cognitive function.

Fasting has also been shown to possibly have beneficial effects on neurological conditions such as Parkinson's disease and Alzheimer's disease.

Delays Aging

While all of the reasons are still unclear to scientists, studies have been clear that intermittent fasting can delay aging and increase lifespan. This has been found true in both human and animal studies. Scientists believe part of the reason may be because of the role fasting plays in the mitochondrial cells and their production, but there is still more to the equation and additional studies are in the process.

Induces Cell Repair

Autophagy is an important role in keeping a homeostatic system. The role it plays is critical, as it recycles old cells that could lead to degeneration, and replaces them with younger and healthier cells. This process is so important for the prevention of disease that scientists are trying to find a way to create a drug that will have the same effect and cross the blood-brain barrier, but as of yet, that is not an option. Thankfully, short-term intermittent fasting has been found to greatly increase this process. One study even found that fasting can shift stem cells from a dormant state to a state of self-regeneration.

May Prevent and Treat Cancer

While the studies are still in the early phases, meaning there are not yet studies on humans, the information out there regarding fasting and cancer is promising. Studies on rats have indicated that alternate-day fasting may stop tumor formation, both animal and test-tube studies have shown it may prevent cancer, and in one test-tube study exposing cancer cells to fasting was as effective as chemotherapy in delaying tumor growth. Fasting was also able to increase the effectiveness of the chemotherapy.

Reduces Oxidative Stress

Oxidative stress caused by free radicals is

extremely damaging to the body and can lead to aging and disease. These free radicals react with healthy cells all throughout our bodies and damage them. Thankfully, multiple studies have shown that fasting can lead to a striking reduction in oxidative stress markers and increase the antioxidant uric acid.

Converts Fats

Not only does intermittent fasting help you lose weight, but a study in mice indicates that it may also turn white fat into brown fat. Believe it or not, fat is not just fat. There are multiple types and some are better than others. White fat is what is commonly accepted as "unhealthy" fat, but brown fat is a much healthier fat that actually helps your body burn off the stores of white fat.

Creates More Brain Cells

Studies have shown that intermittent fasting can increase the rate of neurogenesis in the brain, causing more growth and development of important nerve tissues and brain cells. Higher rates of neurogenesis have been linked to increases in brain performance, mood, memory, and focus. It is able to do this by triggering the brain-derived neurotrophic factor, otherwise known as BDNF. Stimulating this can increase cell growth in the hippocampus, cortex, and basal forebrain, along with other areas of the nervous system.

Increases Energy

Like the ketogenic diet, intermittent fasting also increases the creation of new mitochondrial cells. These cells act as a fuel source for your body, converting food into energy and carrying it the cells that need it. The mitochondrial cell provides ninety percent of the energy your body requires, and boosting the number of cells will boost your energy levels. Not only does it give you physical energy, but mental energy, as well.

Controls Seizures

Intermittent fasting increases the number of ketones in the brain, thus protecting from and preventing seizures. This, alone, is powerful but can be even more powerful on the ketogenic diet for people who have hard-to-control epilepsy.

Boosts Metabolism

Long-term fasting, dieting, and calorie restriction can slow down the metabolism, which already slows with age. On the other hand, regular intermittent fast followed by regular meals can help stimulate the metabolism helping you burn fat more quickly while retaining muscle mass.

Chapter 6: The Fundamentals of Intermittent Fasting

Skipping meals and going a day or two without eating may not seem healthy, but the science speaks for itself. Intermittent fasting, when paired with eating a healthy calorie count when not fasting, has been shown to increase health, weight loss, and prevent disease. In this chapter, we will go over the fundamentals of intermittent fasting and how you can get started. It may be scary, but it can be surprisingly easy, and it only becomes even simpler as you adjust to this way of life.

The Fed and Fasted State

To understand how your body responds to fasting, it is important to first understand how the fed and fasted states work.

The fed states begin when you eat, and typically last for three to five hours, as your body digests and absorbs the food and nutrients. When in a fed state it is difficult for your body to burn any adipose, otherwise known as body fat because your insulin levels are high and it is trying to burn off what you just ate.

After the three to five hour fed state, your body will go into a post-absorptive state. This state simply means that your body is no longer digesting a meal, your insulin levels are low, and it is easier to burn fat. This state tends to last eight to twelve hours.

A fasted state typically does not start until twelve hours after you have eaten a meal, and in modern society, it is uncommon for our bodies to be in this state. Many people will lose weight without much effort when intermittent fasting even if they don't change what they eat, how much they eat, or how often they exercise, because when in a fasted state, your body easily burns your adipose tissue or the stored fat.

It may seem unhealthy and unnatural to fast, after all, how is it different from starvation? The difference is that fasting is intentional, meaning you can do it in healthy ways so that you still get all of the nutrients your body requires. There is nothing negative about waiting to eat between dinner and breakfast; in fact, it has been shown to be better for your health to have the break between meals. Yet, breakfast is named for "breaking fast", meaning you have been fasting overnight and are breaking the fast by eating your morning meal. There is nothing unhealthy or unnatural about this, and similarly, intermittent fasting can be done in a healthy and balanced way.

Life is about balance, and this means that it is neither unhealthy avoiding eating nor binge eats all the time. Intermittent fasting is about finding the balance your body needs in order to receive all of the vital nutrients and calories it needs, but with still receiving all of the health benefits your body can get by taking breaks from digestion.

12/12

The 12/12 method of intermittent fasting is arguably the easiest method of scheduled fasting. For this method, you simply adhere to a 12-hour fasting window and a 12-hour eating window. This plan is easier for beginners, as the fasting window is relatively small, and much of the fasting can be done while sleeping. This plan gives you the benefit of having a more flexible schedule, will give you the ability to still enjoy plenty of delicious and nutritious food daily, and it will cut down on cravings. One of the easiest ways in which to do this plan is to fast from 7 pm and until 7 am.

16/8

The 16/8 is one of the most common intermittent fasting methods. The 16/8 can also be referred to as the Leangains diet, and it is as simple as fasting for a sixteen-hour window and eating during an eight-hour window. This method is fasting is great for people who did not find much help from the twelve-hour fast, or for those who would like to challenge themselves a bit more.

While anyone can do this fast, sometimes men will choose to fast for a full sixteen-hours and some women will choose to fast for fourteen-hours. Typically people will finish their evening meal no later than 8 pm, and then will skip breakfast the next day, not eating again until noon.

One study on mice found that limiting their feeding window to only eight hours protected the mice from obesity, inflammation, diabetes, and liver disease, even if the mice at the same number of calories as mice that ate however much they pleased.

This type of intermittent fasting can because a very easy habit to develop. People naturally fall into eating schedules where they eat meals at the same time every day, and it is the same with this type of fasting. Once you are adjusted to it, it will feel easy, natural, and won't take much thought. All you have to do is learn to not eat at specific times of the day.

Meal Skipping

Meal skipping is easily the simplest way to fast without worrying about being hungry, fitting it into your schedule, or feeling tired. For meal skipping, you simply skip a meal when you are not hungry and wait until the next meal time to eat again. This method is great for beginners or people with time constraints. It is important to note that this method will not have as many health or weight loss benefits, and it is important to eat healthy meals that are not overly calorie dense when you do eat.

Meal skipping is most likely to be successful when the person listens to their body and does it when they are not feeling hungry rather than forcing themselves to fast, otherwise, they are more likely to overeat later in the day. This method may feel more natural and be less stressful for people, especially those new to fasting.

2 Days Every 5 Days

People who are following a 5:2 diet, or otherwise eating standard amounts of healthy food five days a week and fasting two days a week, do not fully give up eating on the two fasting days. Typically, men will consume about 600 calories on fasting days while women will consume 500 calories. The fasting days are also typically separate so that you are not fasting two days in a row. For instance, you could fast on Tuesdays and Thursdays, so that you get plenty of healthy calories and nutrients in on Wednesday.

The research regarding this type of fasting is limited, although it was found that it leads to a similar amount of weight loss as calorie restriction, but without having to restrict calories on the five eating days. This type of fast specifically has been shown to reduce insulin levels and improve insulin sensitivity.

Weekly 24-Hour Fast

Fasting completely, with no calories in-between, once or twice weekly is known as the Eat-Stop-Eat diet. This fast is made easier by not starting at the beginning of the day but in the middle. You can start this fast after either breakfast or lunch, and follow the fast until the same time the following day. This way you are not hungry or tired, but you are still getting a full twenty-four-hour fast. During the fasting period, you can still have water, tea, and other calorie-free drinks.

Eating should be resumed to normal on non-fasting days to ensure getting enough calories and nutrition in. It may be difficult to do a full twenty-four-hour fast if you are struggling to try a shorter fast first. On the other hand, a longer fast such as this is easier when paired on a ketogenic diet, as your body is already in ketosis and burning fats and ketones for fuel, meaning you will be less hungry and tired.

Alternate Day Fasting

There are multiple forms of alternate day fasting, a type of fast which involves the person, obviously, fasting every other day. Some people on alternate day fasting will choose to not eat anything at all on their fast days, while others will allow up to 500 calories. On non-fast days people will often eat as much as they please.

A study on alternate day fasting reported that it was effective for weight loss and heart health, both in overweight and healthy individuals. The participants were able to lose on average just over eleven pounds in a twelve week period.

Alternate day fasting is rather extreme and difficult for many people; it may not be safe for beginners or those with severe medical conditions. It may also be hard to maintain long-term and discouraging for beginners. It is recommended that if you want to try this method of fasting, that you first are experienced with shorter and easier fasts.

Warrior Diet

The Warrior Diet is a more extreme form of intermittent fasting. A person on this method of fasting may eat very little, just a few servings of raw fruits and vegetables, during their twenty-hour fast. At night the person then eats one really large meal, with an eating window of four hours. This method of fasting is best for people who have already tried intermittent fasting and are up to a challenge.

During the eating window, people should make sure to eat large amounts of vegetables, proteins, and fats, along with small amounts of carbohydrates.

Some people struggle to eat such a large meal at night, close to bedtime, and there is a risk people may not eat enough fiber or other nutrients, which would increase health complications.

Advocates for the Warrior Diet claim that humans have naturally been nocturnal eaters through history and that eating at night will allow the body to gain more nutrients due to the circadian rhythm.

Busting the Myths

Myth: Eating frequently is better for the metabolism.

Truth: The myth of eating many small meals throughout the day instead of a few large meals is said to boost the metabolism. This myth has been repeated so frequently so that it is now believed to be fact, but the truth is that it has no scientific backing. The reason this myth began is that each time you eat the metabolic rate does increase slightly for a few hours, though it then takes energy to break down and absorb the food as more energy. This process is known as the thermic effect of food. The amount of energy your body expends in proportional to the number of calories and nutrients that were consumed during your meal.

To explain how the thermic effect works, let's measure the effect of 2,500 calories over the span of a single day, both with smaller meals and larger meals.

Example 1: Six small meals of 416 calories each.
Example 2: Three medium meals of 833 calories.
Example 3: Two large meals of 1,250 calories each.

Your metabolism will increase with all three of these examples, thanks to the thermic effect of food. Although, it will change slightly depending on which of the above meals you are eating. Example one will result in a very weak boost to the metabolic rate that comes and goes frequently throughout the day. Whereas, example three will result in a larger and longer boost that only gradually tapers off. Example two will be somewhere between these two methods.

None of the above examples is superior to another. At the end of a twenty-four-hour period, or however long it takes to process and absorb all of the nutrients, there is no difference in the thermic food effect. The total amount of energy your body has expended is identical in each of the examples, and you are unable to 'trick' your body into burning more calories by manipulating how frequently you eat.

Scientific studies and reviews have found that any evidence of a metabolic boost from more frequent meals is at best very weak. In fact, there are many studies that refute that there is any difference in metabolic rate depending on the size and frequency of meals.

Myth: Eating frequent small meals to control hunger.

Truth: There are surprisingly few studies

done on meal size and the correlation to hunger. Nevertheless, current research that includes meal patterns and protein intakes closest to most peoples' eating habits indicates that appetite control is superior when eating fewer larger meals.

What affects the appetite more than meal size is the nutrient source of the meal. You can eat one thousand calories of ice cream and be hungry again in an hour or two. Yet, if you eat one thousand calories of a nutritionally balanced meal that is high in fat and moderate to high in protein, such as a ketogenic meal, you can feel satisfied half of the day. This is even more effective when you have been on the ketogenic diet for more than a few weeks and are keto-adapted, as your body is used to using fat and ketones as fuel and will keep you fuller for longer.

Myth: Eat small meals to control blood sugar.

Truth: It is commonly claimed by dietitians and health "experts" that eating smaller meals throughout the day will provide you with a stable energy source, prevent hunger pangs, and keep your brain sharp and focused. This is believed to be due to the effects of blood sugar. Contrary to popular belief, in healthy people, blood sugar is actually quite well controlled. Unless you are eating highly unbalanced meals, such as bowls of ice cream, your blood sugar is not likely to spike up and down throughout the day. Going a few hours without food, or even a full day, is not going to make a healthy person's blood sugar drop.

Maintaining blood sugar is a high priority of the human body, and due to this, we have efficient pathways that will keep it stable, even under extreme conditions. Studies show that even if you were to fast for 23 hours and then go on a ninety-minute run, your blood sugar would not drop. It would take at least three days of fasting in order for your blood sugar to drop enough to affect you mentally, and by that point, your body will adjust and start fueling off of ketones in place of glucose. One study revealed that even after fasting for two full days, the blood sugar is maintained steady within normal ranges and cognition levels were not negatively affected, either.

While correct that blood sugar does affect hunger, "low" just means "lower range" in healthy people, and when their blood sugar is signaling to eat, it is not an actual low. More important than blood sugar, is your regular meal patterns, which affects the hormone ghrelin and other metabolic hormones. The release of ghrelin will make people extremely hungry and likely to eat much more than they otherwise would. When you eat at irregular intervals each day, the secretion of ghrelin will not be well controlled making you more likely to overeat. The cells that produce ghrelin have a circadian clock that synchronizes in the anticipation of food with metabolic cycles. This means, that if you set up regularly scheduled eating times that your body will adjust to you eating at those times and you are less likely to feel hungry at other times, as long as you ate the appropriate amount of calories and nutrients.

Myth: Fasting causes the body to go into starvation mode.

Truth: Through human history efficient adaption to a famine has been important for survival. The metabolic rate lowers during starvation, allowing us to live longer and giving us the possibility of finding something to eat. Starvation is completely different from fasting. Skipping a meal or not eating for a twenty-four hour period will not cause the human body to go into this starvation mode.

One study showed that a drop in metabolic rate as a result of fasting only occurs after sixty hours minimum. In that study, the drop resulted in an eight percent decrease in the resting metabolic rate. Other studies did not show an impact in the metabolic rate until between seventy-two to ninety-six hours.

On the contrary, fasting frequently increases the metabolic rate, some studies showing an increase of 3.4%-10% after thirty-six to forty-eight hours. Therefore, short-term fasting, or fasting lasting less than sixty-hours, can increase the metabolic rate and improve weight loss.

Myth: The body only absorbs thirty grams of protein at a time, so you should spread out meals.

Truth: The myth of only being able to absorb thirty grams out of any given meal most likely started due to a misunderstanding of a scientific study from 1997. This study showed that thirty-grams of whey protein got absorbed over the span of three to four hours. People most likely misunderstood this study, thinking that protein could only be absorbed thirty grams at a time and that in order to stay in an anabolic state that they would, therefore, have to eat protein again every three to four hours.

If you think about this in a historical context, you can see that this would have greatly impacted human survival, if it were the case. Humans would not have been able to keep up with the protein demand.

The truth is that the more protein you eat the longer it takes in order to be digested and utilized. A meal of pizza at 600 calories, 75 carbohydrates, 37 grams of protein, and 17 grams of fat is still not fully digested after five hours, and the amino acids are still in the process of being released into your bloodstream and absorbed into the muscle. This is despite pizza being a refined food high in glucose, which is absorbed quickly compared to most foods.

This means that a large steak with a large serving of vegetables and butter would take well over ten hours to digest. The speed of digestion and absorption greatly varies depending on the type of meal and nutrients you are eating and what you have previously eaten in the day. The speed of digestion and protein absorption into muscle can vary greatly, but you will absorb all of it, just slowly over time.

Myth: Fasting causes muscle loss.

Truth: While it is important to eat, on the ketogenic diet, it will not use the gluconeogenesis process to convert your lean muscle mass into glucose. That does not mean intermittent fasting will lead to muscle loss. Protein, or rather amino acids, is absorbed into the body at a very slow rate. This means that if you eat a high protein meal such as a steak with vegetables and butter with dinner with some cottage cheese and berries for dessert, you can consume about one hundred grams of protein, which will slowly be digested and absorbed over a period of somewhere between sixteen to twenty-four hours. This is a common type of meal for someone on the ketogenic diet or a 16/8 fasting period and will not only provide plenty of protein but other nutrients, as well.

This slow period of digestion and absorption means that even if you are not eating, your body is still being provided with protein from the meal you ate before beginning your fast.

As long as you are not fasting for over twenty-four hours, then you should have no problems with the gluconeogenesis process causing lean muscle mass loss.

Myth: Breakfast is the most important meal of the day.

Truth: The act of skipping breakfast is associated with higher body weight. The reason for this is simple, it is because people who skip breakfast are more likely to be dieting in a haphazard manner or eating recklessly. The first set of people follow crash diets, which often result in later on gaining even more weight back, or failing and binge eating when they becoming overly hungry. The second set of people are often living life on the run, and end up grabbing doughnuts or candy bars later in the day, or grabbing fast food take-out for dinner.

Most of the people who skip breakfast are not someone who reads about the details of nutrition and eats regular balanced and nutritious meals, which is why breakfast is associated with a higher body weight.

People will sometimes make an argument for eating breakfast saying that we are more insulin sensitive in the morning. While this is true, that is because people are always more insulin sensitive after a fast, and going all night without eating is a short fast. Insulin sensitivity is always increased once glycogen has been depleted; it is not that breakfast has extra nutritious properties. Even if it did, as long as you are following the ketogenic diet and fasting regularly, your insulin sensitivity should already be optimized.

Myth: Fasting increases cortisol levels.

Truth: Cortisol is the stress hormone, although, it does more than just raise stress levels. Cortisol plays an integral role in blood pressure, the immune system, and breaking down protein, glucose, and fats. Cortisol has gotten a rather bad reputation in the fitness and health communities, but we have this hormone for an important reason. A peak of cortisol helps us get out of bed in the morning; if we didn't have it we would be lethargic and depressed. Elevated levels of cortisol aid us in exercise, by helping increase our performance, mobilize fats, and increase the endorphins post workout.

While chronically high levels of cortisol cause long-term stress and depression, we can't do without spikes in cortisol. We need a balance proportion in our system.

Cortisol levels typically follow a rhythm each day, where they peak in the morning and decline in the evening. While studies of fasting during Ramadan have shown a change in cortisol levels, the change is simply in the rhythm the cortisol goes through during the day. The average level of cortisol over a twenty-four-hour period remains unchanged.

People worry that fasting will increase cortisol and therefore cause problems in muscle tone, but, a study on rugby players during Ramadan also proved this to be false. During the study, despite training, while dehydrated and without either a pre-workout or post-workout protein intake, the players were able to lose fat and retain muscle.

Myth: If you exercise while fasting you'll be weak and lose muscle tone.

Truth: There is a large body of research on sports and fitness performance during Ramadan and it concludes that aerobic exercises, such as an hour of running, have a small but significant impact on performance. The reason for this is largely dehydration. If you are staying well hydrated, you are much less likely to experience problems.

The studies that are more accurate as to intermittent fasting are ones that are not during Ramadan so that the participants are fully hydrated. These studies show that strength and lower intensity endurance training is usually unaffected, even after three days of fasting. Some types of training are decreased without glucose, and in this case, it would improve your results to follow the targeted ketogenic diet and begin your fast after your workout.

Put simply, exercising will not cause loss of muscle tone, and while you may choose to exercise while fed, it is not detrimental to train while fasting.

Myth: Eat a large breakfast and a small dinner.

Truth: While people believe that eating larger amounts of food later at night leads to weight gain, there is not any scientific evidence to support this belief. A large reason why eating late at night is believed to cause weight gain is because this late night eating is often snacking on unnecessary calories or unhealthy junk food. There are no studies showing that a larger evening meal results in negative body composition.

On the contrary, numerous studies on fasting during Ramadan show that a regular nightly feast has either a neutral or a positive effect on body fat percentage and overall health. This is an extreme example, which is especially telling. During Ramadan, people will literally gorge on carbohydrates and treats during the middle of the night, and to no ill effect.

If that isn't enough to convince you, there are plenty of other studies on weight loss that show no weight gain from eating later in the day. One study compared a group eating most of their calories early in the day while another group ate most of their calories late in the day. The group who ate more in the morning lost more weight, but the extra weight they lost was muscle tone. The group that ate more calories in the evening conserved more muscle mass and lost more body fat.

Chapter 7: Combining Intermittent Fasting and the Ketogenic Diet

Intermittent fasting doesn't have to be difficult, especially when paired with the ketogenic diet. When you are in ketosis, your body is used to using ketones as fuel and going for long periods without eating, making the transition from eating days to fasting days much easier. Not only does the ketogenic diet make fasting easier, but they both have many of the same benefits that can work together and strengthen each other. The ketogenic diet combined with intermittent fasting is even more powerful, and vice-versa.

More Manageable Fasting

There is little point in intermittent fasting if you end up having intense hunger cravings, stress, and end up caving and binge eating whatever you can get your hands on. Intermittent fasting is supposed to be a simple and natural process. The ketogenic diet helps out, as your body is already in ketosis and being fueled off of fats and ketones. You shouldn't have any, or at least many, hunger pangs or cravings while intermittent fasting, as long as you are keto-adapted.

Being in the process of ketosis means that along with not feeling hungry, that intermittent fasting will feel more natural. You may begin intermittent fasting without even thinking about it because you will be so satisfied with a meal that you won't need to eat for a very long time.

Pairing the two also lessens any other symptoms. When going on a longer fast, such as a twenty-four or forty-eight hour fast, people can develop headaches and fatigue from their bodies needing to adjust to the lack of glucose in their system. On the ketogenic diet, you have already adjusted to not having glucose and glycogen stores, it won't be much different from what your body is already used to, cutting down greatly on side effects.

Enter Ketosis Sooner

Some people choose to push their body into ketosis more quickly when starting out on the ketogenic diet. They do this in order to shorten the dreaded keto flu and become keto-adapted sooner. While many people prefer to hold off on fasting until after they are keto-adapted, if you are someone who would like to have a slightly harder beginning in order to cut down on the length of time, then this option may be for you.

If you would like to enter ketosis sooner start

by eating a ketogenic meal as low in carbs as you can possibly make it. You will want to include plenty of healthy fats and protein to sustain you over your first fast. After you eat your meal, start a twenty-four-hour fast. The following two days after your fasting, continue to keep your carbohydrate count as low as possible.

After the initial first two days after your fast, you can proceed to eat the normal ketogenic carbohydrate recommendation, which is on average twenty-five to thirty net carbohydrates. The fast will be a more intense beginning to the ketogenic diet, but it is a great way in order to reach ketosis quickly. If you start on a Friday night you should have the worst of it over before work on Monday morning.

Lose Weight Faster

One of the most common reasons for people to

turn to both intermittent fasting and the ketogenic diet is for weight loss. Living with a slow metabolism, or after years of crash dieting, many people struggle to get rid of the extra weight. Both intermittent fasting and the ketogenic diet can help aid weight loss, and when paired together the results are even more amazing.

Some of the reasons for this are:

- When you limit your eating window, you are eating all of your day's calories in a shorter span of time, and this prevents you from being able to eat as much since you will be too full.

- You don't snack. Unnecessary snacking, whether from hunger or boredom, can cause quite a spike in a day's calorie intake. Removing this from the equation can greatly increase weight loss. You can eliminate unneeded snacking both by limiting the eating window and by being full and satisfied for longer periods from the ketogenic diet.

- Less binge eating. Think about a day of dieting. You start out the day highly motivated, but after a stressful day of work and too little to eat, you are hungry and just don't care about dieting anymore, so you eat. A lot. It is all too common for people to fall off the wagon when dieting and end up eating even more calories. The ketogenic diet prevents this when intermittent fasting by keeping you satisfied with long-burning fats and proteins.

Create a Self-Healing Environment

Intermittent fasting activates the cellular cleaning process autophagy. This phenomenon causes the body to literally recycle its own cells. In the process, autophagy removes harmful and toxic compounds and creates healthier younger cells. Different processes of autophagy happen on two conditions:

- One, when the body is being fasted or starved.
- Two, when proteins and carbohydrates are restricted.
-

When you are on both, the ketogenic diet and intermittent fasting, both of these things are happening at once, meaning you can reap all of the benefits from this process. You will not only receive more benefits, but you will do so in a healthy and efficient manner.

Boost Your Brain

The brain is one of the largest consumers of energy out of everything in the human body. Ketones are not just a more efficient energy source than glucose; they are a healthier energy source, as well. Not only does the increase in ketones protect your brain from aging and neurodegenerative diseases, but it will also give you more mental energy, focus, and the list of benefits goes on.

Combining the ketogenic diet with intermittent fasting will cause your ketone level to go up much higher than either of them alone could; boosting the benefits you receive, as well.

Burn More Fat

When you are on the ketogenic diet, you burn more body fat as you don't have glucose and stores of glycogen in your liver and muscles. Your body can hold about two-thousand calories worth of glucose and glycogen at any given time, and when you aren't storing that you switch from burning calories to burning body fat much quicker.

When you are fasting, you burn off body fat even more quickly, as you don't have any calories in your system. If you are an athlete you may consider saving fasting for after your training sessions, but if you are just trying to lose weight and maintain health then exercising while fasting can be a fantastic boost to your metabolism and weight loss.

Spend Less Time Cooking

One of the biggest complaints people have when it comes to eating healthy is not having enough time to cook food. While it is possible to get some healthy ketogenic options on the go, the options are more limited and they still are not as healthy as homemade options. Thankfully, the ketogenic diet paired with intermittent fasting greatly cuts down on cooking time, and can even save you money. Imagine just having to cook one or two meals a day, and if you plan ahead of time you can spend one evening a week cooking a couple of different meal options that you can eat throughout the week. No more daily cooking, no more hassle, but all of the health benefits.

Reduce Inflammation and Oxidative Stress

Two things that worsen diseases are inflammation and oxidative stress. Inflammation is supposed to be a part of a healthy immune system, but all too often with chronic illness, it increases to levels where it not only causes severe pain but worsens the symptoms of the illness as well. Oxidative stress is something everyone has, whether chronically ill or not. Oxidative stress, caused by free radicals, is a flaw in the human system where free radicals cause dangerous cell damage.

Not only does the ketogenic diet and intermittent fasting help reduce inflammation and oxidative stress, but they can also even prevent them. Alone, the ketogenic diet and fasting can have a powerful effect, but the healing properties of them are even more dramatic when paired together.

Energy Boost

Are you tired of always being tired? Are you living life one cup of coffee to the next? Surviving off of energy drinks? Living in an exhausted fog? You are not alone. Between always living life on the go, the high density of unhealthy food, and the rate of chronic illness, many people have a difficult time just waking up in the morning or getting through the afternoon.

Both the ketogenic diet and intermittent fasting helps control insulin and blood sugar, along with providing your body with longer burning fuel, which will keep you energized and moving with fewer energy crashes.

Ketones, fats, and proteins are much slower burning fuel sources than glucose. When you are eating a carbohydrate-heavy diet, your body will go through energy crashes every few hours, whenever you burn off the glucose you have digested. This sends you through an energy roller coaster that is anything but fun.

Detox

We all have days where we want to "cheat" on our diets. Whether it is for a holiday, birthday, or wedding, sometimes we want to enjoy a slice of our favorite cake or go out for some pizza and drinks with friends. Having a fast after indulging allows your body to rid itself of the glucose stores, along with any harmful processed sugar and chemicals. Fasting causes your body to go into a healing and cleansing mode, helping you recover from junk food, sugar, stress, lack of sleep, air pollutants, and more.

When you are on a standard western diet it may be difficult to fast after a cheat day or holiday, but when you are on the ketogenic diet your body is already adapted and can handle it without difficulties.

Intermittent fasting may feel uncomfortable in the beginning, but give it some time to adjust. The longer you are on the ketogenic diet, the more natural it will feel, the less hungry you will be, and the longer you will be able to fast for. The ketogenic diet and intermittent fasting will be like second nature before long, and you will continue to reap the benefits.

Chapter 8: Common Mistakes and How to Avoid Them

When adjusting to a new way of life, it is easy to make mistakes. In this chapter, we will discuss the most common mistakes made on both the ketogenic diet and intermittent fasting, so that not only can you combat and fix these mistakes, but hopefully avoid them altogether.

Obsessing over the Scale

Many people can lose four pounds or more on their first week of the ketogenic diet or intermittent fasting. These results are great and encourage many people to start out, to take a chance and give it a go. The problem is that some people may not see the scale move as much, and become discouraged.

Different people lose weight differently, but just because the numbers on the scale may not be moving does not mean the ketogenic diet and intermittent fasting isn't working. Some people it just takes a little more time, due to illness or a history of crash dieting.

While the scale may not be moving, you are still likely losing fat in vital places. Along with weighing yourself, try measuring your bust, chest, waist, hips, midway between hips and thighs, thighs, knees calves, upper arms, and forearms. Write these measurements down and track them weekly. Many people will lose inches in these places, despite the scale staying still.

If you are still discouraged from tracking your measurement then try tracking them biweekly or bimonthly, rather than once a week.

Not Eating Enough

If you want to lose fat, it is important to eat fat on the ketogenic diet. The basic principle of the ketogenic diet is that you get approximately seventy percent of your day's calorie intake from fat. You don't have to worry about this being too much fat because fat is not what causes you to gain body fat.

It is imperative to get enough fats and calories; otherwise, you will develop deficiencies and unhealthy eating habits. Along with fats make sure you are eating a variety of low-carbohydrate fruits and vegetables, and healthy sources of protein. Try to vary your protein sources, so that you are getting a healthy combination of beef, chicken, lamb, eggs, shrimp, fish, organ meats, etc.

When intermittent fasting, you naturally eat less, yet it is important to make sure you fully reach your calorie goals when you are not fasting, to enable yourself to get all the nutrition you need and fuel to energize your brain and other cells.

Getting Dehydrated

Dehydration is a common problem on the ketogenic diet and intermittent fasting, as your body is dumping excess glucose and glycogen, which attach the water molecules. Even if you are drinking the same amount of water, as usual, your body will be dumping more, making you dehydrated. This can lead to headaches, constipation, fatigue, dry skin, muscle cramps, kidney stones, dry mouth, bad breath, and more. Water is essential to living.

To stay hydrated be sure to keep a bottle of water with you at all times. There is an abundance of reusable water bottles on the market, which makes taking water with you on the go simple.

If you dislike drinking unflavored water you

can always add lemon juice, make tea sweetened with SweetLeaf stevia drops, ketogenic electrolyte packets such as Ultima Replenisher, or sugar-free and artificial sweetener-free flavorings such as Stur Water Enhancer.

Not Sleeping Enough

Not getting enough sleep or having a disorder of the circadian rhythm can decrease energy and make weight loss more difficult. When you don't get enough sleep the body produces less of the human growth hormone, your glucose metabolism is impaired, leptin hormone levels are decreased, and ghrelin levels are increased.

Leptin is an important hormone in order to feel satisfied and full after a meal, and ghrelin is a hormone that tells the body you are hungry. When these hormones are off balance you can constantly feel hungry, leading to overeating and stress.

Try to ensure you get between seven and eight hours of sleep every day, try to not eat a heavy meal within three hours of bedtime, don't exercise within three or four hours of going to bed, avoid using electronics late at night, and sleep in complete darkness for the best sleep.

Not Knowing Your Macros

Calories count, even when you are eating a low-carbohydrate ketogenic diet. Although, when you are eating high fat, moderate protein, and nutritious foods you naturally will not be as hungry and therefore are unlikely to eat too many calories.

This does not mean eating a low-carbohydrate diet will guarantee weight loss. The closer you are to your goal weight, the more time and more difficult it will become, and you will have to pay even closer attention to your macros. Use a ketogenic macro calculator online or on an app to ensure you are eating the proper proportions of fats, carbohydrates, and proteins.

Not Eating Enough Protein

Eating sufficient amounts of protein is extremely important, especially for those on the ketogenic diet and who are practicing intermittent fasting. This is because if you are not eating enough protein your body will begin to convert lean muscle mass into glucose.

Eating sufficient levels of protein can also help you break through a weight loss plateau. When you eat a meal that is high in protein your body will release the hormone glucagon, which assists in counterbalancing insulin and can have an instrumental role in satiety.

This does not mean you should over-eat protein, but ensure that it consists of twenty to twenty-five percent of your daily calorie intake.

Avoiding Vegetables

When trying to keep carbohydrates low many people forsake vegetables and fruits, which is a mistake as they provide nutrients and health benefits that incredibly important. Low-carbohydrate fruits and vegetables have a very important place in the ketogenic diet and intermittent fasting lifestyles. Try to enjoy large quantities of low-starch fruits and vegetables such as broccoli, cauliflower, cabbage, zucchini, bell peppers, green beans, avocados, berries, and more.

Obsessing over Ketone Levels

People are often confused over their ketone levels. Either the person doesn't understand why they aren't losing weight despite high ketone levels, or the person is concerned because their ketone levels are not as high as they would like. There is no reason to worry.

While you can track your ketone levels with urine strips, it is not needed. Having a higher level of ketones does not increase weight loss. Your ketone levels may decrease over time, but as long as they are above 0.5 you are still in ketosis.

The reason the ketone levels will decrease over time is that the longer you are in ketosis the more your body adapts, and it learns to make the number of ketones you need without excess so your body will not be dumping large amounts through urine. The only reason to desire increasingly high ketone levels is if you have a condition such as epilepsy or Alzheimer's disease where the ketones protect the brain from the disease. In this case, you can add exogenous ketones to your diet to increase the number and the neural benefits.

Too Many Nuts and Too Much Dairy

Many people make the mistake of eating nuts and dairy, which in turn causes their weight to stall. A person could potentially even gain weight by eating too much of these items, even while fasting and on the ketogenic diet.

Eating too many nuts, while healthy and great in small portions, could potentially kick someone out of ketosis. This is because they are calorie dense and extremely easy to overeat. One-hundred grams of macadamia nuts contains just over seven hundred calories and over seventy grams of fat, which for most people trying to lose weight is half of their calorie intake.

Nuts are a great source of healthy fats, insoluble fiber, and they don't affect the blood sugar. You shouldn't try to avoid nuts altogether unless you are allergic. Just be sure to enjoy them in moderation.

Similarly, full-fat dairy is also high in calories and easy to overeat. You are also unable to eat reduced-fat dairy on the ketogenic diet, as it is higher in carbohydrates. Another aspect of dairy that makes it tricky in high servings is that it contains a type of protein that leads to greater increases in insulin spikes than other types of protein.

If dairy is causing your insulin to spike or you are having an unexplained weight loss plateau, try to cut down on the number of dairy products such as cheese and yogurt. Cream and grass-fed butter are low in protein, making them a safer option when you are struggling with weight loss.

Eating Low-Carbohydrate Treats

There are some delicious low-carbohydrate baked treat options, and it can be easy to eat plenty of them. These are not a good option for those just starting out on the ketogenic diet. While delicious, they are often high in nuts, and even the ones that aren't will still increase cravings and appetite levels, making it more difficult to eat the appropriate amount and fast. When starting out on the ketogenic diet and intermittent fasting, or trying to lose weight, it is best to avoid these baked goods. Save them for when you are trying to maintain weight. If you have a sweet tooth it is better to reach for a fat bomb or a piece of sugar-free dark chocolate, such as Lily's dark chocolate bars and chips.

Avoid processed foods that are labeled as "low carbohydrate". These items are often high in carbohydrates than they seem and have deceptive labeling. Eat real food rather than anything processed.

Drinking Alcohol

Alcohol is not a good option for those on the ketogenic diet and intermittent fasting, especially when trying to lose weight. Aside from adding unhelpful calories, alcohol is disadvantageous to weight loss. Even when consuming alcohol without carbohydrates, your body is unable to store alcohol as fat, meaning it must metabolize alcohol before anything else. This means that your body is unable to metabolize anything else until the alcohol has been fully processed. Alcohol can also cause dehydration, increased hunger, and lack of self-control, none of which are helpful for weight loss.

Alcohol will also convert to acetate, making breathalyzer ketone trackers inaccurate.

Not Planning

Multiple studies have shown that planning, tracking, and community support can all significantly improve your weight loss and help you reach your goals.

Plan your meals in advance as it will help prevent excessive snacking, binge eating, and grabbing something that isn't as healthy of a choice. You won't have to track your diet forever, but tracking, in the beginning, can help you avoid mistakes while you adjust to the new lifestyle or find any problems if you are having a weight loss plateau.

Cheating

While people on the cyclical or targeted ketogenic diet may enjoy higher carbohydrate meals, this does not mean you should eat "cheat" foods. Foods such as junk food, sugar-laden desserts, anything fried in vegetable or peanut oils, these are all unhealthy options that don't count as a carb-up meal.

It is okay to allow yourself cheat days from

time to time, such as on your birthday or a favorite holiday, but if your goal is weight loss then you don't want to engage in frequent cheat days.

Too Much Snacking

When following a nutritious ketogenic diet, you should not need a snack, unless you have hypoglycemia. Three large meals, or even less, should be more than enough for a single day. If you are struggling with hunger between meals, try these tricks:

- Do not eat unless you are hungry; even if that means you skip meals. Once you are fully keto-adapted and intermittent fasting this will be more likely, and it is perfectly healthy to have a spontaneous fast by skipping a meal.

- If you find that you are in need of snacks, it means your meals likely were either not nutritious enough or were not large enough. Try to increase portion size, include plenty of fiber from fresh fruits and vegetables, and a moderate to a large serving of protein.

- Ensure that you are eating "real" food such as eggs, fatty fish, meat, healthy fats, non-starchy vegetables, fermented foods, and healthy dairy options.

Not Exercising

Many people don't exercise when fasting out of fear that there may be negative consequences, but studies have shown that it is perfectly safe. In fact, you will notice even more results from exercising while fasted than you otherwise would, especially regarding fat loss. Since your body does not need to burn off can digested food it can focus all of its energy on burning off stored adipose tissue, also known as body fat.

If you are struggling with a weight loss plateau, then try adding in a regular workout while in a fasted state and you are more likely to reap the benefits.

Doing Too Much Too Soon

If you are a person who is used to eating every few hours or always eats first thing in the morning, then you should give your body time to adapt before going on a long fast. While it is possible to start out the ketogenic diet by pushing yourself into a quick ketosis with a twenty-four-hour fast, many find a twelve-hour fast easier to start out on. A simple twelve-hour fast may not be as effective, but with it, you won't be as hungry or stressed. A twelve-hour fast is most often easiest when it begins at 8 PM and goes until 8 AM so that you sleep through most of it without hunger cravings keeping you awake at night.

You can then gradually increase your fasting

window by thirty minutes every two to three days until you reach your goal.

The same is true of your exercise routine. While your body is adjusting to the change in diet and fasting you may need to ease up slightly on your workout, so that it does not strain your body as much. Each week you can add a bit of intensity until you meet or exceed your usual time-span or intensity.

The key to starting out on the ketogenic diet and intermittent fasting is to be patient. It may take time to adapt, but if you are patient the process will be easier.

Giving Up

Intermittent fasting and the ketogenic diet take some discipline, especially in the beginning. The first week is the most difficult, but afterward, each week gets easier. You may feel hungry, develop headaches, and crave all of your favorite foods. This will pass. If you stick with it, even just for two weeks, then you will come out on the other side, not only happy that you made the change and feeling much better, but you will be proud of yourself.

Chapter 9: Planning for Success

Going into the ketogenic diet and intermittent fasting without a plan is a sure way of setting yourself up for failure. Before you start to weigh and measure yourself, find a collection of tasty looking recipes, plan out your week's menu and if you have the time you can even cook meals ahead of time to keep in the fridge.

There are many reasons to plan ahead, but one of the biggest reasons is because if you know what you are going to eat and have taken steps to make it available, then when you are fasting and are hungry, you don't have to worry about not knowing what to eat during your eating window.

Start out your diet, or even each week, with a plan such as the following:

Sunday:
- Fast until noon.
- First Meal: Eggs with cheese and an avocado, along with a side of berries.
- Second Meal: A large steak with butter and sautéed mushrooms with a large Cobb salad.

Monday:
- First Meal: Bulletproof coffee and sliced ham.
- Second Meal: Egg salad lettuce wraps, sliced cucumbers, and walnuts.
- Third Meal: Spaghetti squash with marinara sauce, beef meatballs, olive oil, and cheese.

Tuesday:
- Fast until noon.
- First Meal: Roasted salmon with butter and capers and Brussels sprouts with bacon.
- Second Meal: Pork chops with butter

and green beans topped with bacon and chopped pecans.

Wednesday:
- First Meal: Frittata and coffee.
- Second Meal: Japanese stir-fry with beef and sesame oil.
- Third Meal: Pizza made on a fat-head or cauliflower crust, with your favorite low-carbohydrate toppings.

Thursday:
- Fast until noon.
- First Meal: Eggs, roasted tomatoes, asparagus, and fried bacon.
- Second Meal: Lettuce wrapped cheeseburger.

Friday:
- First Meal: Mushroom and cheese omelet.
- Second Meal: Cheesy tuna salad with celery.

- Third Meal: Broccoli cheddar soup with chicken tenders.

Saturday:
- Fast until noon.
- First Meal: Cottage cheese, berries, and almonds.
- Second Meal: Taco salad with beef, lettuce, sour cream, guacamole, onions, and salsa.

After you plan out what days you want to fast on and what meals you plan to eat during the week, you can decide if you want to cook any food ahead of time and make an exercise schedule. If you are just starting out, try to schedule your workouts while feeding. Later on, as you adjust to the ketogenic diet and intermittent fasting, you can purposefully workout while fasting so that you will burn even more body fat, but it is best to allow yourself to adjust first.

Jimmy Clark

Chapter 10: Possible Side Effects

While studies show that the ketogenic diet and intermittent fasting are safe, when using the guidelines outlined in this book, there are still possible side effects. Most of the side effects that are likely to go along with both the ketogenic diet and intermittent fasting, since they both cause the ketosis process. In this chapter, we will go over the most common side effects, their causes, and how you can combat them for the easiest process possible.

Headaches

Probably the most common side effect people complain of is pounding headaches. These commonly start within a day or two of starting the ketogenic diet or a fast and can make it a struggle to go about your daily life. In order to cut down on the effect it could have on the work week, many people start the ketogenic diet or their first fast at the beginning of the weekend. If started on Friday evening, you may still have a headache sticking around by Monday morning, but it will be much milder and easy to handle.

Most of these headaches are caused by the same factors, which are dehydration, electrolyte imbalance, sugar withdrawal, and metabolic confusion.

There is little that can be done about sugar withdrawal and metabolic confusion, you have had to give your body time to process the change and adjust. The other two, dehydration and electrolyte imbalance, are easy to handle with water, nutrients, or put the two together and try out a keto-approved electrolyte drink, such as Ultima Replenisher.

Dehydration

When you are starting out on your ketogenic and fasting lifestyle your body will flush large amounts of water and electrolytes as it dumps glycogen stores from your body. This can lead to dehydration and symptoms such as headaches, constipation, muscle cramps, weakness, and brain fog.

While a common problem, dehydration is simple to fix. Common recommendations are to drink half of your body's weight in ounces. If you weigh one hundred fifty pounds then you would need to drink seventy-five ounces of water a day, though more could be better to fight off dehydration. When drinking large amounts of water, be sure that you don't drink more than a liter of liquids an hour, as your body is unable to process any more of that in such a short span of time.

Electrolyte Imbalance

Electrolyte imbalances go hand in hand with dehydration. This is because when the body dumps large amounts of water, it is also dumping electrolytes, and whenever you hydrate if you do not adequately refuel on electrolyte they will become diluted.

Refueling on electrolytes is extremely important, as they are chemicals in the body that form electrically charged particles in fluids. They then carry the electrical energy needed for many functions such as muscle contractions and nerve impulse transmission.
To keep your electrolytes balanced, to try to consume about five thousand milligrams of sodium a day, along with four hundred milligrams of magnesium and three thousand milligrams of potassium.

Fatigue

Along with headaches, fatigue is one of the

most common problems when beginning the ketogenic diet or intermittent fasting. Thankfully, over time it seems to work itself out, as it is most often caused by the change in diet. Once your body adjusts to the change then your energy levels should increase, until you have even more energy than you did on your previous diet.

If you would like to increase your energy levels in the meantime, then you can try consuming more MCT oil. MCT, otherwise known as medium-chain triglycerides, is a type of shorter chain fatty acid that is more quickly digested. Instead of going through a very long digestion process like most fats, they are able to go straight to the liver in order to be sent throughout the body aiding in energy.

Malnutrition

While the ketogenic diet and intermittent fasting should be healthy at their core, people do not always succeed in keeping their diet balanced. This is a common problem because people are either afraid of the carbohydrate count in vegetables, even in low-starch and keto approved vegetables, or because the person uses a 'lazy' method in which they consume large quantities of processed foods packaged as "low-carb" instead of vegetables.

To ensure you have a healthy diet, make sure to not only focus on your macronutrients such as fats, proteins, and carbohydrates but also on micronutrients, such as vitamins and minerals. Try to eat nutritionally balanced whole foods.

Brain Fog

Brain fog is when your brain feels slow and as if it is filled with sludge, making doing anything, even thinking, difficult. This symptom is often caused by high levels of ammonia and depressed levels of GABA.

While ketosis can increase brain health and function, reducing levels of brain fog, the process of adjusting the ketogenic diet and intermittent fasting may cause an increase in brain fog, until you adapt. To decrease brain fog try to stay hydrated, consume electrolytes, perform light exercises, and eat regularly until you adjust.

Hunger

High levels are known to cause stress, agitation, and weakness. To reduce the likelihood of hunger, try to only eat when you are hungry because if you begin to eat when you are not hungry, it will affect the ghrelin hormone, which tells your body to eat. Over time this hormone will begin to think you need to eat at certain times of the day, even if you do not.

To prevent hunger while fasting, it can be

easier to adapt to the ketogenic diet before you begin fasting so that your body will more efficiently run off of ketones, fats, and proteins. When starting out on intermittent fasting it can also be easier to start with a short fast and gradually increase the length as you adjust.

Kidney Stones

Kidney stones are formed when there is an increase of crystal-forming substances such as uric acid, calcium, and oxalate. While kidney stones are painful, they can typically be avoided by healthy individuals as long as proteins are kept in overall moderate amounts and you stay hydrated.

If you are someone who is prone to kidney stones then doctors have found an effective prevention and treatment that may help you. Consuming a potassium citrate supplement will help reduce the frequency by adjusting the acidity levels of urine, making the kidneys rid themselves of the uric acid that most often causes kidney stones.

Another option for potassium citrate is lemon juice. While not as effective, the natural citrate found in lemons has been shown to help prevent kidney stones in a similar manner. Try adding lemon to your drinking water, or make a sugar-free lemonade with lemon juice and stevia sweetener.

Insomnia

Insomnia can have many causes, whether chronic or acute. Some of these causes may include stress, depression, hormonal changes, hunger, substance abuse, medications, sleep apnea, and stimulants such as caffeine, chronic illness, and lifestyle changes. When beginning the ketogenic diet and intermittent fasting, many people develop insomnia and are unable to pin down the cause.

Insomnia can have a largely detrimental effect on daily life, on both your work and social life. Thankfully, while chronic insomnia may be more difficult to treat, acute insomnia tends to be simpler.

The two most common causes of insomnia on the ketogenic diet and intermittent fastings are the keto flu and hunger. There is nothing you can do for the keto flu itself, aside from treating the symptoms of dehydration and by adding in moderate exercise.

People who have adjusted to intermittent fasting do not tend to be hungry during a fast, but you may when you begin. To reduce the likelihood of it affecting your sleep, try to either fast during the day instead of at night, or try fasting after a large evening meal that should keep you satisfied throughout the night. You will want to ensure the meal has large amounts of fats, moderate to large amounts of protein, and is highly nutritious.

Sometimes high-fat meals can also interfere with sleep. It does this because fats are a long-burning and high energy source, and if your body has not adjusted to this newfound energy you may be unable to sleep. To prevent these many people will try to not eat within three hours of bedtime.

Lastly, try to not exercise or drink any stimulants within three hours of bedtime, and try to avoid electronic lights, such as computers or phones within an hour of bedtime.

Bad Breath

During the beginning stages of the ketogenic diet, many people experience a bad breath that has a funky fruit smell. This is caused by high levels of the ketone acetone in the body, which are being expelled through the breath. Large amounts of protein, causing an increased amount of ammonia, can also cause bad breath.

There is little you can do to help with bad breath, aside from mouthwash and breath mints, but if the cause is caused by the beginning stages of ketosis, do not fear, it will not last. The ketone acetone, while high in number during the beginning of ketosis, decreases over time and is replaced by more effective ketones.

If you are experiencing bad breath despite being on the ketogenic diet for more than two or three weeks, then watch your protein levels and make sure they do not exceed twenty to twenty-five percent of your day's overall calorie count.

Muscle Cramps

Muscles cramps are common on the ketogenic

diet and intermittent fasting because they go hand in hand with dehydration and electrolyte imbalances. While muscle cramps can have multiple causes, these two are the most common.

If you are following the advice earlier in this chapter on staying hydrated and consuming electrolytes and are still finding yourself with muscle cramps, then there are still options. Try to increase your magnesium levels with magnesium supplements, Epsom salt baths or foot soaks, or Epsom salt muscle gels.

Digestive Problems

One of the most common causes of people giving up on the ketogenic diet is stomach upset. Symptoms such as diarrhea, gas, cramps, and constipation may be common when starting out on the ketogenic diet, but they do not tend to last long. The most prominent trigger for stomach upset is dehydration, candida die-off, and lack of fiber, too much MCT oil, and metabolic confusion.

There is little you can do about metabolic confusion, but this is also an easy case, as it will go away on its own. Once your body adjusts to the change in diet, after a few weeks, digestive problems should go away.

Many people will develop constipation, as a result of having fewer carbohydrates and therefore less fiber in their diets. This is easy to manage, just try to ensure that you eat plenty of sources of keto-approved fruits, vegetables, and nuts.

If you suspect that you might have a high candidacy for it, cut off sugar, and try to increase fermented foods in your diet. Foods such as kimchi and homemade yogurt are great choices.

Large amounts of MCT oil may also cause a

variety of symptoms of stomach distress. This is because unlike other fats, MCT oil is digested extremely quickly and if your body is not adjusted to a high-fat diet, it is easy to have negative side effects. Try cutting back a bit on the MCT until your body adjusts to your new lifestyle.

Sugar alcohols are great sweetener option on the ketogenic diet, because they have zero net carbohydrates, as the body does not process them. However, this aspect of sugar alcohols may also cause stomach pain and diarrhea. To avoid this, try to only consume erythritol, as it is the type of sugar alcohol known to cause the least amount of negative side effects. Try to keep how much you eat limited, as well. Erythritol seems to be well tolerated in moderate quantities, but high amounts may still cause unpleasant effects.

Hair Loss

Any significant diet change, whether intermittent fasting, the ketogenic diet, or any other diet, may possibly cause some people hair loss. Small amounts of hair loss usually occur within three to six months of the diet change. While unwanted, it is usually only minimal amounts of hair loss, and it soon grows back as thick as ever.

To keep any hair loss to a minimum, and hopefully prevent it altogether, ensure that you are not eating too large of a calorie deficit. This can be easy when intermittent fasting, but it is important to not only eat enough calories for your body type and activity level but to eat plenty of vitamins and minerals, as well. While you may want to lose a lot of weight quickly, it is better for your body to lose weight gradually over time. You are also more likely to keep the weight off if you take your time instead of rushing the process.

One study has shown that a common cause of hair loss on the ketogenic diet is from people overly limiting their protein intake. Ensure that twenty to twenty-five percent of your daily calorie intakes are from protein, otherwise, you likely will develop negative side effects. Try to spread your protein out throughout your meals of the day, as well, instead of including them all during one meal.

While any large stress or change in life can cause hair loss, you may consider adding in a multivitamin that contains iron, zinc, and biotin.

Elevated Heart Rate

Some people may develop a racing heart rate, known as tachycardia, or heart palpitations during the ketogenic diet and intermittent fasting. If you start experiencing problems, you should see your doctor and get checked out to make sure it is not a serious unrelated condition. Thankfully, when it is caused by the diet change, it is most often caused by dehydration and a lack of sodium. Try to increase your water and sodium intake and it should go away.

If you are chronically ill or have any health conditions, you should work along with your doctor to ensure that your change in diet is safe for you.

Ketoacidosis

While ketosis is a perfectly safe state in which your body is producing ketones to use as fuel in place of glucose, the state of ketoacidosis is not safe and is in fact life-threatening. Thankfully, most people on the ketogenic diet do not have to worry about developing ketoacidosis.

Studies have found that even people who are at a heavyweight and fasting for long periods do not develop ketoacidosis unless they have an underlying health condition.

Ketoacidosis is caused by people, whose pancreas is malfunctioning, preventing an insulin response from stopping too many ketones from being produced. If too many ketones are created, then the blood will become acidic. This is why it is incredibly important for anyone with diabetes, especially type I diabetes, to work in conjunction with their doctors when going on the ketogenic diet or considering fasting.

If you are concerned that you may be developing ketoacidosis, then it is important to go to the ER immediately. Watch for symptoms such as shortness of breath, extreme thirst, vomiting, confusion, dehydration, and stomach pain.

Reduced Exercise Performance

Athletes are often concerned about how a lifestyle change may affect their performance. This is a valid concern; especially as in the beginning stages of the ketogenic diet and intermittent fasting are likely to reduce your stamina and strength.

During the first month of fasting and in the process of adjusting to ketosis, your body is trying to adapt, it does not yet know how to use ketones and fat as effectively as it used glucose. Thankfully, this is only during the short-term.

Long-term the ketogenic diet and fasting have been shown to increase performance, or at the very least not negatively impact it. If you are currently in the season of your activity that requires more workouts and stamina than usual, it is best to hold off on fasting and the ketogenic diet until the off-season. Try to start the process during the month that you have the least amount of commitments for your sport or activity. It can also help if you allow your body to adjust to the ketogenic diet before you add in fasting.

Many athletes choose to try the targeted or cyclical ketogenic diets, as these are geared towards people with high-intensity workouts that require a lot of strength and stamina. However, it is best to start out on the ketogenic diet and only adjust it to the cyclical or targeted versions after you have been on the diet for four to six weeks and your body has fully adjusted to the process of ketosis.

Likewise, save your fasting for when you are not training or performing in your sport.

Chapter 11: Frequently Asked Questions

In this chapter, we will go over questions frequently asked about the ketogenic diet and intermittent fasting to help you get well on your way to success.

Is There a Better Time of Day to Fast?

Some people believe that the warrior's diet fast is more in tune with human nature and history, providing extra benefits by fasting in the day and eating at night. Some studies do support that there may be some benefit to this, but it is still inconclusive. As there is currently no hard evidence, it is best to fast whenever it fits best into your lifestyle and preferences.

Do I Start Counting My Fast After Completing the Meal or After the First Bite?

A fast contains no eating; therefore, you fast will not begin until after you have finished every bite of a meal.

Will I Lose Muscle Tone If I Practice Intermittent Fasting Long-Term?

While it is possible to lose muscle tone with any fasting or dieting, if you practice intermittent fasting correctly you will not lose any muscle tone. In order to keep your muscle tone, it is important to eat plenty of protein when you are not fasting. Eat moderate amounts of protein on non-fasting days, and before you start a fast eat a high-protein meal.

Does 20 Calories of Cream in My Coffee Hurt?

While most people suggest consuming nothing containing calories, it technically does not count as breaking your fast as long as you consume no more than fifty calories during the fasting period. This does not mean you can have fifty calories worth of cream in your coffee three times during your fast. But, you can allow yourself to have fifty calories worth spread throughout your fast.

Should I Still Fast If I'm at My Goal Weight?

While fasting and the ketogenic diet are great for weight loss, they have many health benefits besides those regarding your weight. If you are at your goal weight, just make sure that you are reaching your full calorie recommendation. This means if your calorie intake is supposed to be sixteen-hundred calories and you fast until noon, that you will want to consume all of those calories regardless, to keep on the weight.

Do I Have to Fast Every Day or Is It Okay to Miss Some Days?

There is no need to fast daily. While some people choose to do so, it is much more common to fast every other day or only a couple of days a week.

Is There Any Way to Not Skip Breakfast If Get My Daily Energy from It?

While most people find fasting during the morning, and thus skipping breakfast, easier and more natural, there is no need to fast specifically in the morning. Fast whenever you feel like it! You can start your fast directly after breakfast if you like.

How Long Is It Safe to Fast For?

Studies have found fasting up to seventy-two hours to be generally safe. However, it generally is not recommended to fast for this length of time for intermittent fasting. Remember, intermittent fasting is about repeated short fasts. Generally, you will probably want to keep your fasts to a maximum of twenty-four hours. You don't want to fast that is overly long, because with intermittent fasting it becomes a lifestyle, and you want a lifestyle that you can maintain while still getting proper levels of nutrition and calories.

Will I Be Hungry While Fasting?

You may be hungry at first, but you don't have to be. You can start out by eating a large filling meal full of fats and proteins before your fast and then start with short fasts. Every few fasts try adding an additional thirty minutes in length until you get to your goal. Slowly starting your fast like this can keep you from being hungry, as you are allowing your body to adjust slowly at its own pace.

How Long Does It Take to Get into Ketosis?

The length of time it takes to get into ketosis varies from person to person, and it changes based on what your usual diet is, what the last meal before you started fasting or the ketogenic diet, and whether or not you are starting out the ketogenic diet with a fast. On average it takes two days to a week.

Can I Drink While Fasting?

Yes, you can drink! It is important to stay hydrated. While people don't drink during fasting during Ramadan, that is for religious reasons, not health reasons. You are allowed any non-caloric drinks that don't contain any artificial sweeteners.

Can I Take My Medicine While Fasting?

By all means, please take any medication. In fact, you should discuss this with both your doctor and your pharmacist. As long as your medications are safe to take while fasting, then proceed to do so. If your medication requires you to have meals prior to taking the medicine, then try to time your fast after you take your meds.

Why Do I Get Cold While Fasting?

Studies show that fasting will increase blood flow to body fat in a process known as adipose tissue blood flow. When fasting, more blood flow is traveling to your adipose tissues, presumably to help it move to your muscles for fuel, vasoconstriction can occur in your toes and fingertips to compensate.

Is Intermittent Fasting Safe for Women?

There are those who will caution women against intermittent fasting, saying that it will negatively impact fertility. This can be true, but only in certain circumstances.

All of the studies that show a negative impact on fertility are for alternate day fasting, not for once or twice weekly fasting. In fact, no study shows that fasting once or twice a week may have a negative impact on women's fertility. On the contrary, while there are some studies showing alternate day fasting having negative female fertility side effects, there are many other alternate days fasting studies on women that show no negative side effects whatsoever.

Some studies even found that despite the metabolic change occurring during intermittent fasting, the ones that are as long as seventy-two hours seem to have no effect on menstrual cycles for people with a normal weight and cycle. Though, it has been found that fasts longer than seventy-two hours may affect the menstrual cycle of people who are extremely underweight.

If you are worried about intermittent fasting throwing off your hormones, then start small. Try out fasting just once or twice a week, and start with a simple twelve-hour fast.

Will I Have Cravings?

Cravings are common in the first month, but by the end of that time most people don't have any cravings, and if they do they are infrequent and easy to manage.

Is the Ketogenic Diet Safe on the Kidneys?

Some people are concerned that high levels of protein may be dangerous to the kidneys.

There is no need to worry about high-protein levels on the ketogenic diet; the recommended protein levels are only moderate, not high. From time to time, you will eat high-protein meals before a fast, but the protein from that one meal is going to slowly be digested over your fast, making it safe.

If you do not have a kidney disease and stay well hydrated, then you should not have a kidney problem with either the ketogenic diet or intermittent fasting.

Will I Feel Tired and Weak?

You likely will feel tired and weak at the beginning of the diet. Although, once you have adjusted to the lack of carbohydrates then you shouldn't feel tired or weak on either the ketogenic diet or intermittent fasting.

Is the Ketogenic Diet a Fad?

No, the ketogenic diet is not a fad. It has been

around for nearly a century for its many health benefits. It is now gaining more popularity since people have learned of its amazing benefits, but it is a long-term solution that works for many people.

Is The Ketogenic Diet and Fasting Safe During Pregnancy or Breastfeeding?

Due to the ethical dilemma, there are no studies on the ketogenic diet and its safety during pregnancy or breastfeeding. It is not recommended, and it is actively recommended for practicing intermittent fasting while pregnant or breastfeeding.

What Is the Difference Between Low-Carbohydrate and the Ketogenic Diet?

A low-carbohydrate diet is simply one that does not contain many carbohydrates, a ketogenic on the other hand is not only low in carbohydrates, but it is also high in fat and moderate in proteins.

How Many Carbohydrates Can You Eat and Still Be in Ketosis?

The number of carbohydrates you can consume will vary depending on your size and activity level. Generally, it is between twenty and fifty net carbohydrates, although it is most often under thirty net carbohydrates.

Is the Ketogenic Diet Safe for Everyone?

The ketogenic diet is extremely safe. The diet has undergone many short-term and longer-term studies that have proven as much. While you may experience some unpleasant side effects, in the beginning, these typically go away within the first month.

Despite the safety of the ketogenic diet, it is

not for everyone. People who are pregnant or kidney disease should avoid this diet. People with diabetes, especially type I diabetes, and other chronic illnesses should be in conjunction with their doctor on this diet, or any other diet, for that matter.

Conclusion

The ketogenic diet and intermittent fasting may be quite a change from what you are used to, but it is a change that will guide you on towards health and your goal weight. Many people, once they have adapted to the change, enjoy eating more than ever, and wouldn't want to go back. Eat less often or eating fewer carbohydrates does not have to mean you are enjoying your food less, but rather more.

Take your time and have patience as you adjust to the process of ketosis. Whether you are beginning the process of the ketogenic diet before you jump into intermittent fasting or decide to dive right into intermittent fasting to kick off the ketogenic diet, it will take patience. The transition to being in a state of ketosis may be difficult at first. Nobody enjoys the flu, even non-contagious and short-lived keto flu. Yet, if you give your body the time it needs to adjust to your new style of eating, you will feel better than ever and before long you will likely be down a pant size.

Thank you for reading Ketogenic Diet and Intermittent Fasting for Beginners: A Complete Guide to the Keto Fasting Lifestyle; Gain the Weight Loss Clarity You Need. I hope you have found it to be a helpful and fulfilling resource that will guide you onto your journey to health and weight loss with whole foods, the ketogenic diet, and intermittent fasting.

www.ingramcontent.com/pod-product-compliance
Lightning Source LLC
Chambersburg PA
CBHW031150020426
42333CB00013B/598